FOGSI Modern Approach to CONTRACEPTION

Series Editor

Hrishikesh D Pai

Editors

Ashish Kale
MD DNB FICOG FICMCH DEPS FICS
Founder Director and Chief IVF Consultant
Department of Obstetrics and Gynecology
Ashakiran Hospital and Asha IVF Centre
Pune, Maharashtra, India

Hrishikesh D Pai
MD FRCOG (UK-HON) FCPS FICOG MSc (USA)
Founder and Medical Director
Bloom IVF Group, Lilavati Hospital IVF Center, Mumbai
Consultant Gynecologist, Lilavati Hospital IVF Center, Mumbai and
Fortis Hospital Bloom IVF Centre, Delhi and Chandigarh
Professor
Department of Reproductive Medicine
DY Patil University
Navi Mumbai, Maharashtra, India
Immediate Past President, FOGSI (2022–2023)
Trustee, FIGO Asia Oceania (2023–2025)
Chief Administrator, FOGSI Manyata Project
Postgraduate Teacher for MD and DNB Courses (1991–2018)

Rishma Dhillon Pai
MD DNB FCPS DGO FICOG
Gynecologist and Infertility Specialist
Department of Obstetrics and Gynecology
Jaslok, Lilavati, and Hinduja Health Care Hospitals
Mumbai, Maharashtra, India

Nandita Palshetkar MD FCPS FICOG FRCOG (UK)
Professor Emeritus
Department of Obstetrics and Gynecology
DY Patil School of Medicine
Navi Mumbai, Maharashtra, India
Infertility Specialist, Lilavati Hospital IVF Center, Mumbai
Scientific Director and Co-Founder, Bloom IVF and BAUFICI Genetics
President, Indian Society for Assisted Reproduction (2022–2024)
President, Association of Maharashtra Obstetric and
Gynaecological Societies (2020–2022)
Past President, FOGSI, IAGE, MOGS and MSR

Sunita Tandulwadkar
MD (Obstetrics and Gynecology) FICS (Gyne-Endoscopy) FICOG
Gynecological Endoscopist and ART IVF Specialist
Chief and Medical Director
Department of Obstetrics and Gynecology, Ruby Hall Clinic
Pune, Maharashtra, India
Chief, Ruby Hall IVF and Endoscopy Center, Pune
Director, Solo Clinic, Center of Excellence Infertility and Endoscopy
Founder and Medical Advisor
Solo Stem Cells, Stem Cells Research and Application Center, Pune
Co-Founder, Solo Research Foundation—Sponsor a Birth
President, IAGE (2019–2020)
Chairperson, Maharashtra Chapter ISAR (2018–2020)

Ashwini Kale DGO DNB FICMCH
Director
Department of Obstetrics and Gynecology
Ashakiran Hospital and Asha IVF Centre
Pune, Maharashtra, India

Co-Editors

Manisha Takhtani Kundnani
MD FNB (Reproductive Medicine) FNUS
Medical Director and Infertility & Reproductive Medicine Specialist
Department of Obstetrics and Gynecology
Fertility Square, The IVF Clinic
Mumbai, Maharashtra, India

Rohan Palshetkar
MS FRM BDRME ADRME
Obstetrician, Gynecologist, and ART Consultant
Professor and Head of Unit, Bloom IVF
Department of Reproductive Medicine
DY Patil School of Medicine and Bloom IVF
Mumbai, Maharashtra, India

Foreword
Hrishikesh D Pai

JAYPEE BROTHERS MEDICAL PUBLISHERS
The Health Sciences Publisher
New Delhi | London

Jaypee Brothers Medical Publishers (P) Ltd.

Headquarters
EMCA House
23/23-B, Ansari Road, Daryaganj
New Delhi 110 002, India
Landline: +91-11-23272143, +91-11-23272703
+91-11-23282021, +91-11-23245672
E-mail: jaypee@jaypeebrothers.com

Corporate Office
Jaypee Brothers Medical Publishers (P) Ltd.
4838/24, Ansari Road, Daryaganj
New Delhi 110 002, India
Phone: +91-11-43574357
Fax: +91-11-43574314
E-mail: jaypee@jaypeebrothers.com

Overseas Office
JP Medical Ltd.
83, Victoria Street, London
SW1H 0HW (UK)
Phone: +44-20 3170 8910
E-mail: info@jpmedpub.com

EU GPSR Authorised Representative
Logos Europe, 9 rue Nicolas Poussin
17000, La Rochelle, France
Phone: +33 (0) 6 67 93 73 78
E-mail: Contact@logoseurope.eu

Website: www.jaypeebrothers.com
Website: www.jaypeedigital.com

Inquiries for bulk sales may be solicited at: jaypee@jaypeebrothers.com

FOGSI Modern Approach to Contraception

First Edition: **2024**

Reprint 2025

ISBN: 978-93-5465-987-4

Printed in India

Dedication

To my patients, staff of Ashakiran Hospital and Asha IVF Centre, and my parents

—Ashish Kale

To my parents Dr Avinash Yelikar and Dr Kanan Yelikar for being the pillar of strength and inspiration and my children Aahana and Aaryan for being patient with me

—Ashwini Kale

CONTRIBUTORS

Apurva S Sholapure
MBBS MS DNB (Obs & Gyne)
Senior Resident
Department of Obstetrics and Gynecology
Government Medical College
Miraj, Maharashtra, India

Ashish Kale
MD DNB FICOG FICMCH DEPS FICS
Founder Director and Chief IVF Consultant
Department of Obstetrics and Gynecology
Ashakiran Hospital and Asha IVF Centre
Pune, Maharashtra, India

Ashwini Kale DGO DNB FICMCH
Director
Department of Obstetrics and Gynecology
Ashakiran Hospital and Asha IVF Centre
Pune, Maharashtra, India

Bhakthraj D Thombre MS
Assistant Professor
Department of Obstetrics and Gynecology
Mahatma Gandhi Institute of
Medical Sciences
Wardha, Maharashtra, India

(Col) Bidhan Roy
MS DNB FGO PGDHHM
Professor and Senior Adviser
Department of Obstetrics and Gynecology
Armed Forces Medical College
Pune, Maharashtra, India

Hafizur Rahman
DNB (Obs & Gyne) DGO FICOG
Additional Professor and Head
Department of Obstetrics and Gynecology
All India Institute of Medical Sciences
Kalyani, West Bengal, India

Indranil Dutta
MBBS MS FICOG FIAOG FIAMS PGDHHM PGDMLS
Professor and Unit Head
Department of Obstetrics and Gynecology
IQ City Medical College
Durgapur, West Bengal, India

Indrani Mukhopadhyay MBBS MS (Obs & Gyne)
Professor
Department of Obstetrics and Gynecology
Armed Forces Medical College
Pune, Maharashtra, India

Jaya Barla MS (Obs & Gyne)
Assistant Professor
Department of Obstetrics and Gynecology
Maharashtra Institute of Medical Education
and Research
Pune, Maharashtra, India

Kananbala Yelikar MBBS MD MICOG FICMCH FICOG
Former Dean
Professor and Head
Department of Obstetrics and Gynecology
Government Medical College and Hospital
Aurangabad, Maharashtra, India
NAAC Coordinator, MEDD

Malavika JC MBBS MS DNB OBG
Associate Professor
SS Institute of Medical Sciences
and Research Center
Davangere, Karnataka, India

(Col) Nagaraja N MBBS MS
Sr Adv (Obst & Gyn) and Trained in ART
Command Hospital (Southern Command)
Department of Obstetrics and Gynecology
Command Hospital
Pune, Maharashtra, India

Poonam Varma Shivkumar MD
Professor and Head
Department of Obstetrics and Gynecology
Mahatma Gandhi Institute of
Medical Sciences
Wardha, Maharashtra, India

Radhika Chetan MBBS MS
Assistant Professor
Department of Obstetrics and Gynecology
Bangalore Medical College and Research
Institute
Bengaluru, Karnataka, India

Ruchika Garg MBBS MD (Obs & Gyne)
Professor
Department of Obstetrics and Gynecology
SN Medical College
Agra, Uttar Pradesh, India

Rupali A Gaikwad MS (Obs & Gyne)
Assistant Professor
Department of Obstetrics and Gynecology
Government Medical College and Hospital
Chhatrapati Sambhajinagar, Maharashtra, India

Sangeeta Tajpuriya MBBS MD FICOG FICMCH
Senior Gynecologist
Department of Obstetrics and Gynecology
Vedansha Hospital
Nagpur, Maharashtra, India

Shobha N Gudi MBBS MD DNB (Obs & Gyne) FICOG
Senior Consultant
Department of Obstetrics and Gynecology
St Philomena's Hospital
Bengaluru, Karnataka, India

Shrinivas N Gadappa MS (Obs & Gyne)
Professor and Head
Department of Obstetrics and Gynecology
Government Medical College and Hospital
Chhatrapati Sambhajinagar, Maharashtra, India

Sivaranjani P MS
Assistant Professor
Department of Obstetrics and Gynecology
All India Institute of Medical Sciences
Kalyani, West Bengal, India

Sonali Deshpande MD (Obs & Gyne)
Academic Professor
Department of Obstetrics and Gynecology
Government Medical College
Dharashiv, Maharashtra, India

Sudesh Doshi
MBBS DGO LLB
Owner–Director
Department of Obstetrics and Gynecology
Agraj Hospital
Solapur, Maharashtra, India

Sushma Sharma MBBS DGO DNB
Professor
Department of Obstetrics and Gynecology
MIMER Medical College and Dr BSTR Hospital
Pune, Maharashtra, India

Swati Badgire MBBS MD (Obs & Gyne)
Assistant Professor
Department of Obstetrics and Gynecology
Government Medical College and Hospital
Aurangabad, Maharashtra, India

Swati Gurav MS DNB MRCOG (Obs & Gyne, London)
Assistant Professor
Department of Obstetrics and Gynecology
BJ Government Medical College
Pune, Maharashtra, India

Uma Wankhede MD (Obs & Gyne)
Professor and Head
Department of Obstetrics and Gynecology
PAH Government Medical College
Pune, Maharashtra, India

FOREWORD

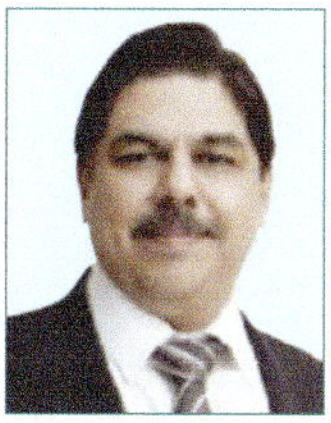

FOGSI Modern Approach to Contraception offers a comprehensive exploration of reproductive health, delving into various facets of contraceptive choices. The table of contents provides a roadmap through the intricacies of contraception, combining guidelines, historical perspectives, and future trends. From traditional methods like male condoms to cutting-edge options such as contraceptive implants and vaginal rings, each chapter is a detailed exploration of effectiveness and application.

Readers will find valuable insights into emergency contraception, medicolegal considerations surrounding sterilization, and specialized contraceptive needs for diverse populations, including transgender individuals. The book extends its focus to safety considerations for women over 35, perimenopausal contraception, and contraception in the context of specific health conditions such as abnormal uterine bleeding, acne, and HIV.

Addressing the continuum of reproductive experiences, the book also covers postpartum intrauterine devices, contraception after abortion or ectopic pregnancy, and guidelines for individuals with HIV and sexually transmitted diseases. Furthermore, the inclusion of the FOGSI-FWC Commitment emphasizes the commitment to quality family planning services in the private sector in India.

FOGSI Modern Approach to Contraception is more than a collection of chapters; it is a guide that navigates the evolving landscape of reproductive choices, offering evidence-based insights to both healthcare professionals and individuals. This book serves as a valuable resource, fostering informed decision-making and contributing to the ongoing dialogue surrounding reproductive health.

Hrishikesh D Pai
President, FOGSI (2022–2023)

PREFACE

"Women have a right to choose
You cannot have maternal health without reproductive health"

Contraception is the basic necessity and need of the hour as India is rapidly inching towards being the most populous country in the world. This book has been launched to address the issues related to contraception of Indian population. To ensure the sanctity of the content, we have roped in seasoned professionals in the field of Obstetrics and Gynecology all over India.

The book also emphasizes on the need of contraception of special age groups and various conditions including teenage and peri-menopausal contraception to cover the whole spectrum of target population. Nowadays, the beneficiaries want a choice of multiple options while deciding the method of contraception. This book will act as a ready-reckoner for practitioners in their day-to-day practice as it covers all the latest evidences and practice guidelines.

This book has multiple chapters on various types of contraception, contraception in special situations leaving no aspect of contraception and family welfare unturned.

Respectful maternity is the right of every female and we must ensure that they are not denied this right. The ability to plan, space and terminate pregnancies are very important aspect of each female leading to a healthy family.

We thank and appreciate all our authors for their contribution. The book has been written in a lucid and comprehensive manner so that the readers enjoy reading it.

Hrishikesh D Pai

ACKNOWLEDGMENTS

We would like to express our sincere gratitude to all those who contributed to the creation of *FOGSI Modern Approach to Contraception*. Special thanks to the dedicated practitioners and experts whose valuable insights and experience enriched the content, making it a comprehensive guide for gynecologists. We extend our appreciation to the contributors who emphasized the importance of addressing diverse needs, covering special age groups and unique conditions in contraception. The commitment to evidence-based information and adherence to the latest practice guidelines are owed to the diligent researchers and professionals involved in this project.

This book would not have been possible without the support from the publishers, M/s Jaypee Brothers Medical Publishers (P) Ltd, New Delhi, India. We wish to acknowledge and thank them for their support. This book stands as a collective effort, and we are grateful to everyone who played a role in its development.

CONTENTS

SECTION 3

GUIDELINES FOR USE IN SELECTED POPULATION

SECTION 1

Overview

CHAPTER 1

Contraceptive Uses: Guidelines and Effectiveness

Kananbala Yelikar, Rupali A Gaikwad

INTRODUCTION

It was in 1952 that India realized the danger of population explosion. The Government of India introduced National Family Planning Program which aimed at population stabilization, ultimately promoting reproductive health, which in turn would help reduce maternal, infant morbidity, and mortality.

The Government of India [Ministry of Health and Family Welfare (MoHFW)] predicted that if the implementation of family planning (FP) is carried out in its proper essence, India could prevent 35,000 maternal deaths and 12 lakh infant deaths. This definitely would result in achieving sustainable development goal (SDG). India has already achieved maternal mortality rate (MMR) of 103 per 1 lakh live births.[1]

The Government of India made newer contraceptives freely available in public hospitals. Injectable contraceptives, centchroman, and progestin-only pills were showed a slow but definite rise in acceptance rate.[2] In 2015, this landmark shift from permanent method of female sterilization to more modern methods created a history.[3]

Oral contraceptives' typical failure rate is 4%. It is safe, effective, and reversible contraceptive. Hence, it is an ideal contraception for delaying, spacing, and limiting births. In spite of being an ideal one, the acceptance rate in India is very low, i.e., only 5.1%.[4]

CONTRACEPTIVE SERVICES UNDER THE NATIONAL FAMILY WELFARE PROGRAM

Spacing methods

- *Rhythm methods:* Calendar method/safe period method/natural method/lactation amenorrhea method (LAM)
- *Barrier methods:* Cervical caps/diaphragms
- *Harmonal Methods:*
    - Combined oral contraceptive (COC) pills (monophasic/biphasic/triphasic)
    - Progesterone-only pills (POPs) (minipills)
    - Postcoital/emergency contraceptive pills
    - Injectable contraception depot medroxyprogesterone acetate (DMPA)
    - Intrauterine contraceptive devices [IUCD—first, second, and third generations—insertion time—postpartum IUCD (PPIUCD), postabortion, interval]
    - Nonsteroidal contraceptive (Centchroman)
    - Subdermal implants
- Vaginal rings (NuvaRing)

Permanent Method

- *Female sterilization tubal ligation:* Minilap/laparoscopy
- Male sterilization (vasectomy).

Types of Combined Oral Contraceptive

Mala N contains levonorgestrel (0.15 mg) + ethinyl estradiol (30 µg). Mala N is supplied free of cost through government health centers and hospitals.

The readily available preparations are given in **Table 1**.

Pharmacology: The usual estrogen component is combined with a different generation of progestin components with varying degrees of androgenic and progestogenic potential **(Table 2)**.

Progestin-only pills' classification according to progestins is described in **Table 3**.

TABLE 1: Combined oral contraceptive pills.

Type of COC	*Preparation*
Monophasic low-dose combined oral contraceptives (COCs)	20–35 µg ethinyl estradiol (EE) and progestogen-like levonorgestrel (LNG)
Biphasic low-dose COCs	Two combinations of estrogen and progestogen, e.g., 7 tablets of 40 µg EE plus 25 µg desogestrel and 15 tablets of 30 µg EE plus 125 µg desogestrel
Triphasic low-dose COCs	Contain the same hormones but in three dose ratios, e.g., 6 tablets of 30 µg EE plus 50 µg LNG, 5 tablets of 40 µg EE plus 75 µg LNG, and 10 tablets of 30 µg EE plus 125 µg LNG
Quadriphasic preparations	Four different combinations of estradiol valerate (EV) and dienogest

USE OF CONTRACEPTIVE

To address women's need for FP, the provision of a wide range of safe, effective, and affordable contraceptive methods is essential. The methods offered must cater to women's needs and preferences.

TABLE 2: Combined oral contraceptive pills.

Estrogen component	*Estradiol, ethinylestradiol, or estetrol*
First-generation progestin	Norethindrone acetate, ethynodiol diacetate, lynestrenol, norethynodrel
Second-generation progestin	Levonorgestrel, dl-norgestrel
Third-generation progestin	Norgestimate, gestodene, desogestrel
Fourth-generation progestin	Drospirenone, cyproterone acetate

TABLE 3: Progestin-only pills (POP) classification according to progestins.

Groups	*Progestins*	*Concentration per tablet*
Continuous administration without pause days:		
POP containing traditional progestins	Norethisterone	0.350 mg 0.500 mg 0.600 mg
	• Norethindrone • Ethinodiol diacetate • Lynestrenol • Norgestrel • Levonorgestrel	0.350 mg 0.500 mg 0.500 mg 0.075 mg 0.030 mg
POP containing desogestrel	Desogestrel	0.075 mg
Continuous administration for 24 days and 4 pause days:		
POP containing drospirenone	Drospirenone	4.0 mg

National Family Health Survey 5 (2019–20) definitely shows a rise in use of modern contraceptives for FP from 47.8% to 56.5 %. Total fertility shows a remarkable decline. The contraceptive prevalence rate CPR) is 67% in reproductive age group. More than 50% married and unmarried women are using modern contraceptives. Female sterilization still remains the most accepted method. Among unmarried sexually active women, male condoms are widely accepted.

Contraceptive use among currently married women rises with[4] number of living children reaching a rate of 80% in multiparous women and employment and socioeconomic statuses. Use of pills, injectables, and condoms is more popular in private sector as compared to sterilizations, intrauterine device (IUD), PPIUCD, and injectables. Emergency contraception still remains an exception.

GUIDELINES

World Health Organization Medical Eligibility Criteria[5]

The WHO medical eligibility criteria (MEC) wheel for contraceptive use has been accepted by the Government of India. The oral contraceptives such as COCs and POPs should be prescribed only in those cases where they fulfill the medical eligibility criteria **(Figs. 1A to C)**. Routine coronavirus disease 2019 (COVID-19) testing is not mandatory before sterilization. Proper assessment of the client, adherence to correct infection prevention, and standard insertion techniques can prevent IUCD insertion-related complications and unnecessary visits to the facility. Postpartum and postabortal phases are most susceptible period for acceptance of contraception.

Effectiveness of Contraceptive[6,7]

Contraceptive effectiveness is described in two ways:

1. *Perfect use:* Pregnancy rates (failure rates) during perfect use show how effective a method is when it is used perfectly, consistently, and exactly according to directions.
2. *Common (or typical) use:* Pregnancy rates (failure rates) during common (or typical) use show how effective a method is during

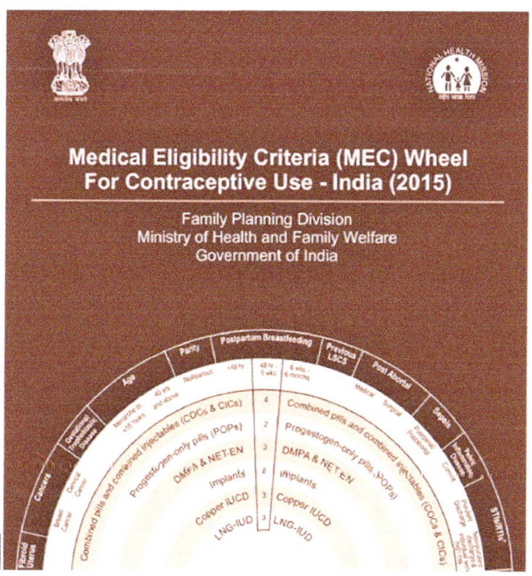

A

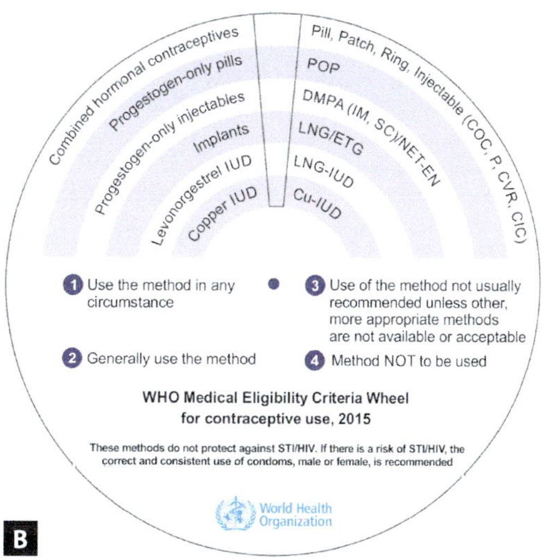

B

Figs. 1A and B

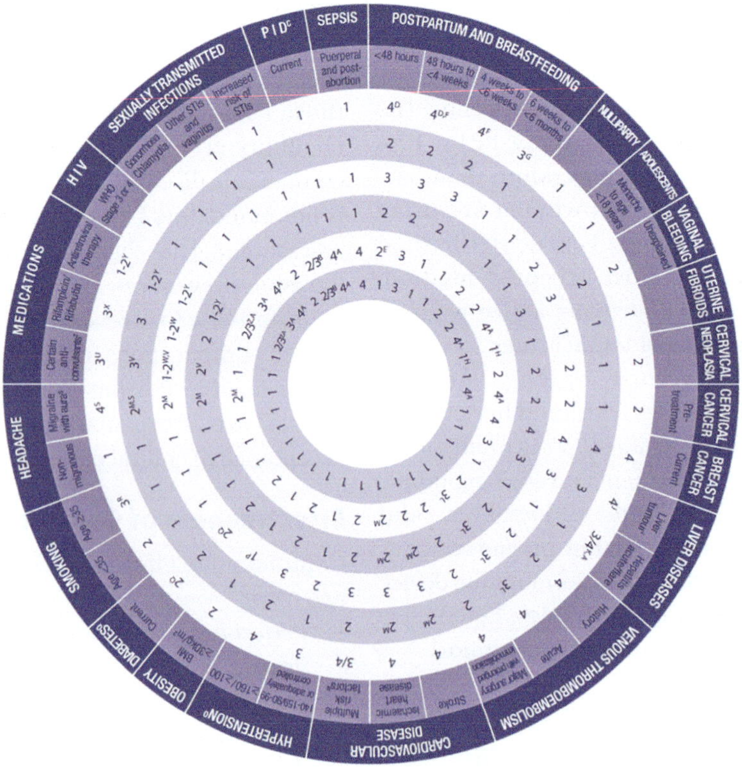

Fig. 1C

Figs. 1A to C: The World Health Organization (WHO) medical eligibility criteria (MEC) wheel.

TABLE 4: Contraceptive effectiveness.

	Contraceptive effectiveness	
Method	***With perfect use***	***With typical use***
COC pills	0.3 pregnancy per 100 women	8 pregnancy per 100 women
POPs	• *Breastfeeding women:* 0.3 pregnancy per 100 women • *Non-breastfeeding:* 0.9 pregnancy per 100 women	*Breastfeeding women:* 1 pregnancy per 100 women *Non-breastfeeding:* 3–10 pregnancy per 100 women
Centchroman (Ormeloxifene)	1–2 pregnancy per 100 women	No documented failure rate with typical use available
Female condoms	5 pregnancies per 100 women	21 pregnancies per 100 women
LAM	0.5 pregnancies per 100 women in the first 6 months after childbirth	2 pregnancies per 100 women in the first 6 months after childbirth

Contd...

Contd...

Method	***Contraceptive effectiveness***
ECPs	ECPs are not a continuous form of birth control; hence, annualized pregnancy rate is not calculated If all 100 women used ECPS containing: • Only progestin, 1 pregnancy per 100 women • Both estrogen and progestin, 2 pregnancy per 100 women The sooner after unprotected sex that ECPs are taken, the more effective they are
Injection DMPA	• The reported first-year failure rate of DMPA is 0.3% • The 2-year pregnancy rate with NET-EN (given every 84 days) was 1.4 per 100 women in contrast to 0.4 women observed for DMPA and NET-EN (given every 60 days) • Pregnancy rate with mesigyna is 0.18 per 100 women years and nil for cyclofem
IUCD	• Pregnancy rates for all major IUDs are less than 1 per 100 women per year • The cumulative pregnancy rate for CuT-380A was 2.1 per 100 women and for CuT-220C was 5.7 • For the LNG-20, a pregnancy rate of 0.3 has been reported after 5 years
Female sterilization	• In the first year after the procedure, there are 0.05 pregnancies per 100 women • Within 10 years after the procedure, 0.75 pregnancies per 100 women • Effectiveness depends partly on how the tubes are blocked

(COC: Combined oral contraceptive; DMPA: depot medroxyprogesterone acetate; ECPs: emergency contraceptive pills; LAM: lactational amenorrhea method; LNG-20: levonorgestrel 20; NET-EN: norethisterone enanthate; POPs: progestin-only pills)

actual use by the average person who does not always use the method consistently and correctly **(Table 4)**.

REFERENCES

1. OCHA. (2014). FP2020 Partnership in Progress 2013-2014. [online] Available from: https://reliefweb.int/report/world/fp2020-partnership-progress-2013-14 [Last accessed January, 2024].
2. Ministry of Health and Family Welfare. Ministry of Health and Family Welfare Initiatives & Achievements-2023. New Delhi: PIB; 2015.
3. Latkin CA, Knowlton AR. Social network assessments and interventions for health behavior change: A critical review. Behav Med. 2015;41:90-7.
4. Ministry of Health and Family Welfare. National Family Health Survey (NFHS-5), 2019-21. Mumbai: IIPS; 2022.
5. WHO. (2015). Medical eligibility criteria wheel for contraceptive use. [online] Available from: https://www.who.int/publications/i/item/9789241549257 [Last accessed January, 2024].
6. IIPS. National Family Health Survey (NFHS) I and II, reports 1992-93 and 1998-99. [online] Available from: https://rchiips.org/nfhs/india1.shtml [Last accessed January, 2024].
7. Family planning division, Ministry of Health and Family Welfare, Government of India. (2016). Reference manual for oral contraceptive pills. [online] Available from: https://nhm.gov.in/images/pdf/programmes/family-planing/guidelines/Reference_Manual_Oral_Pills.pdf [Last accessed January, 2024].

CHAPTER 2

Combined Oral Contraceptive Pills: Past, Present, and Future

Shrinivas N Gadappa, Swati Badgire

INTRODUCTION

Nine percent of currently married women have an unmet need for family planning, down from 13% since 2015-16.[1] The newly developed reversible choices of contraception with improved safety and efficacy have improved women's acceptance to oral combined contraception pills. An oral contraceptive method offers women a variety of choices to delay, space, and to limit births, which is safe, effective, and reversible methods to prevent pregnancy. Combined oral contraception (COC) pill is an integral part of National Family Health Program for contraception. Though, safety and efficacy of COC pills have been proved worldwide, in India, only 5.1% women use COC pills.[1] Among available COC pills, Mala N [levonorgestrel (LNG) 0.15 mg + ethinyl estradiol (EE) 30 µg] is supplied free of charge by Government of India at public health sectors.

PAST OF COMBINED ORAL CONTRACEPTION

Hormonal contraception is in use successfully over more than half a century. In history of pharmacology as well as epidemiology, hormonal contraception represents the most extensively tested chemicals till date. This should not amaze us as contraceptive pills are not meant for treatment of a disease, where side effects if occurred may be expected considering health benefits. In contrast, contraceptive is mainly given to healthy and young woman who do not wish pregnancy at a certain period of time in her life. So, it is obvious that, no woman will take risk to harm their current or later well-being for prevention of pregnancy. That is the main reason, even a rare incident of adverse effect strikes panic which is resolved only years later, either after remodeling of the dose or the launching of new and improved progesterone.

Decrease in dosage of estrogen component has been a major milestone in COCs evolution. These changes were adopted with the intent of improvement in the safety and tolerability without affecting their effecacy.[2] But, the modified low dosage of estrogenic component in COCs is not adequate for persistent inhibition of ovulation. That is why, center of attention has shifted to the progesterone, which is mainly responsible for antiovulatory effects of COCs.[3] In 1980, research has stated that some progesterone may disturb the metabolism of lipids associated with a possibility of increased incidence of arterial diseases.[4] The research has introduced a novel, effective, and "metabolically neutral" synthetic progesterone (norgestimate, gestodene, and desogestrel) which makes contraceptives more safer, although—in 1990s—WHO-sponsored studies stated that these newly developed steroids probably increase the risk of venous thromboembolism in comparison with previous contraceptives containing levonorgestrel (LNG).[5]

TYPES OF COMBINED ORAL CONTRACEPTION

The various preparations of COCs are mentioned in **Table 1**.

TABLE 1: Various preparation of combined oral contraceptions.

Monophasic low-dose	20–35 µg ethinyl estradiol (EE) and progestogen (e.g., levonorgestrel)
Biphasic low-dose	Estrogen and progestogen are combined in two formulations, e.g., first seven pills of 40 µg EE + 25 µg desogestrel and next 15 pills with combination of 30 µg EE + 125 µg desogestrel
Triphasic low-dose	Combination of same harmones with three ratios, e.g., first six pills of 30 µg EE + 50 µg LNG, five pills of 40 µg EE + 75 µg LNG, and 10 pills of 30 µg EE + 125 µg LNG
Quadriphasic preparations	*Combinations of four formulations:* Estradiol valerate (EV) and dienogest

PHARMACOLOGY

Estrogen is combined with a progesterone of different generations with different degrees of androgen and progestogen activity **(Table 2)**.

Efficacy of COCs is reported in two ways. Failure rate is 0.3 pregnancy per 100 women on perfect use, while on common (typical) use, 8 pregnancies per 100 women (HWY).

TABLE 2: Combination of estrogen with a progesterone of different generations.

Estrogen component	Estradiol, ethinylestradiol, or estetrol
1st generation progestin	Ethynodiol diacetate, norethindrone acetate, norethynodrel, and lynestrenol
2nd generation progestin	Levenorgestrel, dl-norgestrel
3rd generation progestin	Norgestimate, desogestrel, and gestodone
4th generation progestin	Drosperinone, cyproterone acetate

MEDICAL ELIGIBILITY CRITERIA (FIGS. 1A AND B)[6]

When to start combined oral contraceptions?

As per wish of a woman for withdrawal bleeding and according to clinical recommendation, prescription can be given as cyclic formulations (21/7, 24/4 cycle), extended cycle formulations (daily pills for 3 months) or continuous use formulations (for 1 year period) **(Table 3)**.

How to use combined oral contraception pills?

One tablet is to be taken each and every day, irrespective of sexual intercourse, till the pack is finished. In 28-tablet packs, soon after finishing the packet, first tablet from the next new packet is to be taken next day. Menses happens when women are on last row pills. Irrespective of bleeding, tablets should be continued.

THE 24/4 REGIMEN: A NOVEL APPROACH TO REDUCING HORMONE FREE INTERVAL

Since its inception, the COCs are being prescribed as a typical 21/7 regime, which comprised of 21 days of active hormones, subsequently followed by a 7-day hormone-free interval (HFI), when a withdrawal bleeding occurs. Evidence shows that 21/7 regimens probably do not sufficiently inhibit

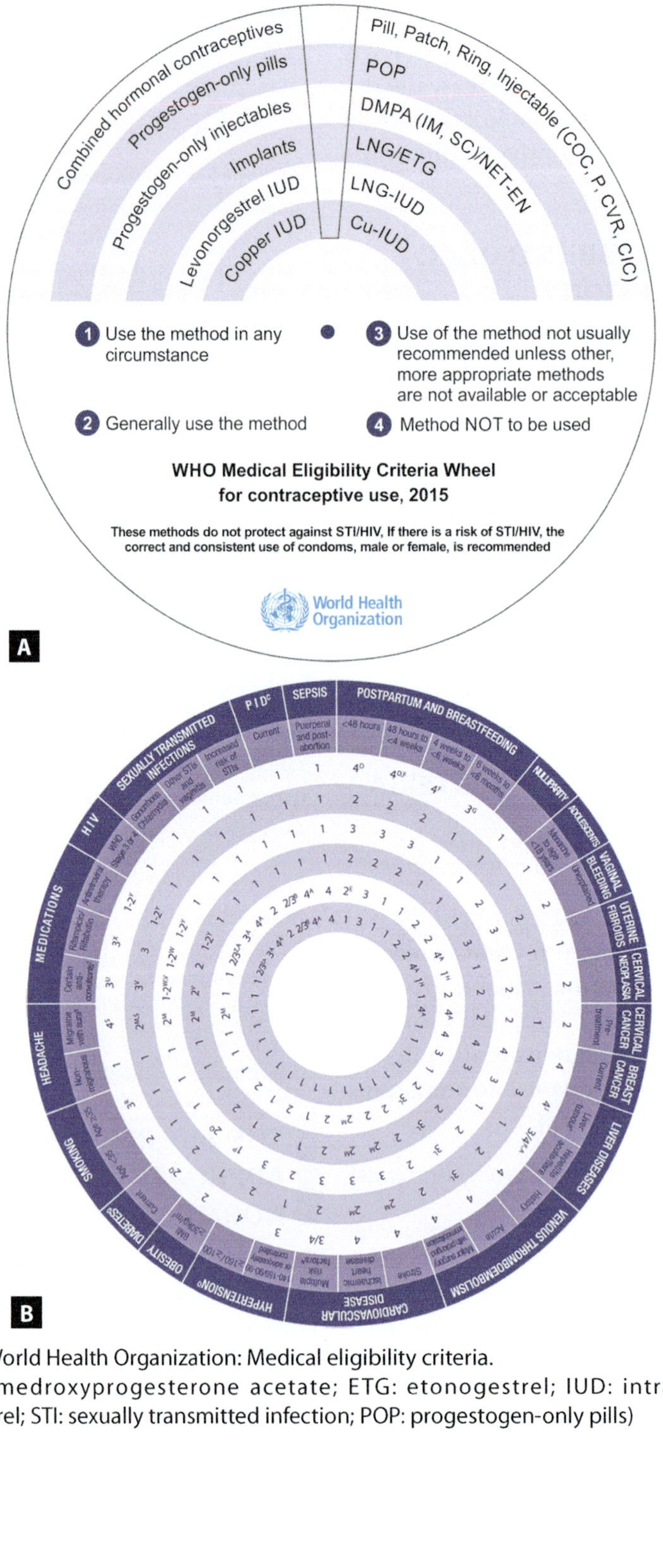

Figs. 1A and B: World Health Organization: Medical eligibility criteria.
(DMPA: depot medroxyprogesterone acetate; ETG: etonogestrel; IUD: intrauterine device; LNG: levonorgestrel; STI: sexually transmitted infection; POP: progestogen-only pills)

TABLE 3: When to start combined oral contraceptive pills.

	Situation	*When to start*	*Back-up method*
1.	Having menstrual cycles	• In first 5 days of menses • After 5th day of menses	• Not required • Required for the first 7 days
Breastfeeding			
2.	• <6 months after giving birth • >6 months after giving birth	• Not recommended • At any time, if her monthly bleeding has not returned. If monthly bleeding has returned (as situation 1)	• Needed for the first 7 days of taking pills
Not-breastfeeding			
3.	• <4 weeks of giving birth • >4 weeks of giving birth	• Any time on days 21–28 after giving birth • Any time, if her menses has not returned • If her monthly bleeding has returned, as per situation 1	• No need • Required for the first 7 days • No need
4.	After abortion	• Within 7 days of abortion • Any time, if ≥7 days and after ruling out pregnancy • In abortion with MMA, it can be started on same day or within 5 days of misoprostol use	• No need • Required in first 7 days • No need
5.	No menses	Any time after ruling out pregnancy	Required for first 7 days
6.	Shifting from a nonhormonal method	• Shifting from Cu-IUD: Within 5 days of menses • If it is >5 days after start of menses	• Not required • Needed for 7 days
7.	Shifting from another hormonal method	• Immediately, if she is a perfect user • At the time of repeat injectable contraceptive	• No need • No need
8.	After taking emergency contraceptive pills	Same day	For first 7 days, back up method is required

(Cu-IUD: copper intrauterine device; MMA: medical methods of abortion)

ovulation.[7] One more major problem is that the HFI causes recurrence of premenstrual symptoms, which are otherwise controlled by active hormonal pills.[8] The highlights of the 24/4 COC regimen are summarized below:[9]

1. Significant inhibition of ovulation.
2. Greater contraceptive safety margin if tablets are forgotten.
3. Prevents hormonal fluctuations that decrease the hormone withdrawal symptoms and improves the quality of life. (4) Advantageous for women who, for various reasons, wish to have a monthly menses.

MANAGEMENT OF MISSING OF PILLS (TABLE 4)

TABLE 4: How to manage forgotten pills?

Forgotten pills	*How to manage*
Forgotten 1 or 2 pills	Take one hormonal tablet as early as possible or take two pills at scheduled time. There is little or no risk of pregnancy
Missed ≥3 days pills in the 1st or 2nd week/ started new pack ≥3 days late?	Take one hormonal pill immediately when she remembers and continue the scheduled pill. A backup is needed for the next 7 days. Also, can consider taking ECPs, if she had sex in the past 72 hours
Missed 3 or more pills in the 3rd week	Take one hormonal pill as soon as possible and finish all hormonal pills in the pack as scheduled. Discard the 7 nonhormonal tablets in a 28-pill pack. Start a fresh pack the very next day. A backup is needed for the next 7 days. Also, can consider taking ECPs, if she had sex in the past 72 hours
Missed nonhormonal tablets	Throw away the missed nonhormonal tablets. Continue COCs one each day. Start fresh pack as usual

(ECPs: emergency contraceptive pills; COCs: combined oral contraceptive pills)

MECHANISM OF ACTION

The main mechanism of action is the prevention of ovulation. Another mechanism is ability of progestin component to thicken the cervical mucus to prevent sperm penetration, slowing tubal motility and delaying sperm transport, and inducing endometrial atrophy.

CONTRAINDICATIONS

Underlying conditions are considered as contraindication **(Table 5)**.

TABLE 5: Contraindications of combined oral contraceptive pills.

Pregnancy	*Uncontrolled hypertension*
Migraine with associated focal neurologic deficit	Thrombophlebitis or thromboembolic disorders
Smokers >35 years of age	History of DVT, thrombotic disorders
Diabetes with vascular involvement	Undiagnosed abnormal genital bleeding
Thrombogenic heart arrhythmias	Diagnosed or suspicion of carcinoma of breast
• Thrombogenic cardiac valvulopathies • Cerebrovascular or coronary artery disease • Hepatic adenomas or carcinomas, jaundice	Carcinoma of the endometrium or other diagnosed or suspicion of estrogen dependent neoplasia

(DVT: deep vein thrombosis)

ADVANTAGES

- *Prevention of pregnancy:* COC pills are one of the most successful means of contraception.
- *Cycle stabilization:* It is a great social advantage for women and is one of main cause of high continuation rate among educated married women.
- *Treatment of menstrual disorders:* COC pills cure dysmenorrhea and ovulation, menorrhagia, and metrorrhagia. It also lessens premenstrual symptoms.
- *Prevention against cancer:* It is one of the most important beneficial effects of COCs. It has been proved that COCs pills directly prevent endometrial cancer and ovarian cancer. It also prevents choriocarcinoma by preventing pregnancy.
- *Protection against benign tumors and related diseases* such as benign breast diseases like fibrocystic and fibroadenomatous

diseases, ovarian functional cysts, and fibromyoma of uterus.

- Protection against diseases such as ectopic pregnancy, pelvic inflammatory diseases, anemia and malnutrition, endometriosis, acne and hirsutism, abnormal uterine bleeding, rheumatoid arthritis, osteoporosis, and premenstrual syndrome.

MINOR SIDE EFFECTS

Minor side effects include nausea, vomiting, and lack of appetite, breakthrough bleeding, oligomenorrhea and amenorrhea, breast changes: Edema of the breast leading to heaviness and tenderness, headache and migraine, chloasma, weight gain, acne, and oily skin, and vaginal discharge.

MAJOR RISKS

Counseling regarding health risks associated with the use of COCs should be done.

- Evidence from observational research states that current users of COC have a 3- to 3.5-fold increased risk of venous thromboembolism as compared to nonusers.[10-12]
- The absolute risk of developing arterial thromboembolism (ATE) in young women is very low, but it increases markedly with age through a woman's reproductive years.[13]
- A recent cohort study stated a relative risk of carcinoma of breast of 1.19 (95% CI: 1.13–1.26) for current or recent users of COC as compared to never-users of hormonal contraceptives.[14]
- An international collaborative epidemiological study of cervical cancer in 2007 stated that current COC use for ≥5 years doubles the cervical cancer risk in comparison with nonuser of COC (RR: 1.90; 95% CI 1.69–2.13).[15]

FUTURE

- *Estetrol-drospirenone combination oral contraceptive:* A natural estrogen and estetrol (E4) is obtained exclusively from the human fetal liver. The E4 used in practice is obtained from plant sources. It has both agonist as well as antagonist properties with a mechanism of action different from SERMs (selective estrogen receptor modulators). This is a potent oral contraceptive with an expected bleeding pattern with low-side effects. Its safety and efficacy are comparable to other available COCs. Phase 4 studies on large scale will be required for confirmation of its efficacy, safety, and adverse event profile.[16]
- *A dual prevention pill (DPP):* It is a daily dose tablet with combination of oral contraceptives and oral preexposure prophylaxis (PrEP). Both components of DPP are approved and licensed nationwide. The DPP is one of the options that could enhance method choice, particularly for women who are already using oral contraceptives. By lifting up the oral contraceptive market and extending to women with an unmet need for contraception, the DPP has the potential to increase the uptake of PrEP.[17]

REFERENCES

1. International Institute for Population Sciences (IIPS) and ICF. National Family Health Survey (NFHS-5), 2019-21: India. Mumbai: IIPS; 2021.
2. Burkman R, Bell C, Serfaty D. The evolution of combined oral contraception: improving the risk-tobenefit ratio. Contraception. 2011; 84:19-34.
3. Guerra JA, López-Muñoz F, Álamo C. Progestins in combined contraceptives. J Exp Clin Med. 2013;5:51-5.

4. Rosenberg L, Palmer JR, Sands MI, Grimes D, Bergman U, Daling J, et al. Modern oral contraceptives and cardiovascular diseases. Am J Obstet Gynecol. 1997;177:707-15.
5. WHO. World Health Organization Collaborative Study of Cardiovascular Disease and Steroid Hormone Contraception: effect of different progestogens in low oestrogen oral contraceptives on venous thromboembolic disease. Lancet. 1995;346:1582-8.
6. World Health Organization. (2015). WHO medical eligibility criteria wheel for contraceptive use–2015 update. [online] Available from: https://www.who.int/publications/i/item/9789241549257 [Last accessed November, 2022].
7. London A, Jensen JT. Rationale for eliminating the hormone-free interval in modern oral contraceptives. Int J Gynaecol Obstet. 2016;134:8-12.
8. Read CM. New regimens with combined oral contraceptive pills moving away from traditional 21/7 cycles. Eur J Contracept Reprod Health Care. 2010;15(Suppl 2):S32-41.
9. Blake J. Evolving Strategies in the Dosing of Oral Contraceptives. Canadian J CME. 2009:35-40.
10. de Bastos M, Stegeman BH, Rosendaal FR, Van Hylckama Vlieg A, Helmerhorst FM, Stijnen T, et al. Combined oral contraceptives: venous thrombosis. Cochrane Database Syst Rev 2014;CD010813.
11. Peragallo Urrutia R, Coeytaux RR, McBroom AJ, Gierisch JM, Havrilesky LJ, Moorman PG, et al. Risk of acute thromboembolic events with oral contraceptive use: a systematic review and meta-analysis. Obstet Gynecol. 2013;122:380-9.
12. Manzoli L, De Vito C, Marzuillo C, Boccia A, Villari P. Oral contraceptives and venous thromboembolism: a systematic review and meta-analysis. Drug Saf. 2012;35:191-205.
13. Lidegaard Ø, Løkkegaard E, Jensen A, Skovlund CW, Keiding N. Thrombotic stroke and myocardial infarction with hormonal contraception. N Engl J Med. 2012;366: 2257-66.
14. Mørch LS, Skovlund CW, Hannaford PC, Iversen L, Fielding S, Lidegaard ø. Contemporary Hormonal Contraception and the Risk of Breast Cancer. N Engl J Med. 2017;377:2228-39.
15. International Collaboration of Epidemiological Studies of Cervical Cancer, Appleby P, Beral V, Berrington de González A, Colin D, Franceschi S, et al. Cervical cancer and hormonal contraceptives: collaborative reanalysis of individual data for 16,573 women with cervical cancer and 35,509 women without cervical cancer from 24 epidemiological studies. Lancet. 2007;370:1609-21.
16. Creinin MD, Westhoff CL, Bouchard C, Chen MJ, Jensen JT, Kaunitz AM, et al. Estetrol-drospirenone combination oral contraceptive: North American phase 3 efficacy and safety results. Contraception. 2021;104:221-8.
17. Friedland BA, Mathur S, Haddad LB. The Promise of the Dual Prevention Pill: A Framework for Development and Introduction. Front Reprod Health. 2021;3: 682689.

CHAPTER 3

Progestin-Only Pills: Past, Present, and Future

Shrinivas N Gadappa, Rupali A Gaikwad

INTRODUCTION

India was the first country in the world to start a National Program for Family Planning in 1952. Over the decades, this program has experienced metamorphosis in numerous ways such as policy and program perpetration. Presently, National Program for Family Planning not only achieve population stabilization pretensions but also promote reproductive health and decrease maternal and child mortality and morbidity.

The Ministry of Health and Family Welfare (MoHFW), Government of India (GOI), estimated that if the current unmet need for family planning is met over the next 5 years, then India could avert 35,000 maternal deaths and 12 lakh infant deaths.[1] In the recently revised World Health Organization's (WHO) Medical Eligibility Criteria (MEC) 2015 for contraceptives, progestin-only pills (POPs) have been moved from category 3 to category 2 for <6 weeks breastfeeding women, which means that they can generally be used in the immediate postpartum period as the advantages outweigh the risks.[2] In India, POPs are currently available for distribution only in the private sector. Taking into consideration the available evidence on the safety, efficacy, and acceptability of the method, the GOI has taken a policy decision to include POPs in an expanded basket of choice for the public health delivery system, which is indeed a step in the right direction.

In 2015, three new contraceptive methods started by the government of India, injectable contraceptive, centchroman, and POPs[3], indicated an important demanded shift from the permanent method of sterilization, which reckoned for two thirds of contraceptives used by Indian population till 2015–2016, to the ultramodern limiting styles of contraception **(Table 1)**.[4]

PAST PROGESTIN-ONLY PILLS

Past POPs were grouped under the name of *traditional POPs*, which offer analogous prospects in contraceptive effectiveness and cycle control also having low inhibitory capacity over ovulation and more specified while breastfeeding. As they are *administered daily and without pause*, their action is to alter cervical mucus and endometrial histology.

ABOUT THE METHOD[5-6]

POPs are also called *mini pills*. They contain lower doses of progestin than combined oral contraceptives (COCs) and prevent pregnancy by thickening the cervical mucus, making it impenetrable to sperm, thinning the endometrium, which makes implantation less likely, suppressing ovulation which is not consistent and happens more likely with desogestrel. It is *essential to have the pill at the same time each day* to maximize contraceptive efficacy, preferably from first day of menses.

TABLE 1: Classification of progestin-only pills (POPs).

Groups	*Progestins*	*Concentration per table*
Continuous administration without pause days:		
	Norethisterone	0.350 mg 0.500 mg 0.600 mg
POP containing traditional progestins	• Norethindrone • Ethynodiol diacetate • Lynestrenol • Norgestrel • Levonorgestrel	0.350 mg 0.500 mg 0.500 mg 0.075 mg 0.030 mg
POP containing desogestrel	Desogestrel	0.075 mg
Continuous administration for 24 days and 4 pause days:		
POP containing drospirenone	Drospirenone	4.0 mg

POPs are safe in breastfeeding women as they will not affect quality and quantity of milk. Bleeding pattern changes are common but not harmful. *Back up contraception* is needed at least for 2 days *if the pill is started >5 days from onset of menses*, or taken *>3 hours late or missed on any given day.*

EFFECTIVENESS

Progestin-only pills may not be as effective as COCs in preventing pregnancy due to lower dose of progestin; there is reliance on mechanisms other than ovulation inhibition and consistent timing is important for effectiveness. Failure rates are <1 pregnancy per 100 women in first year among breastfeeding women, 3–10 pregnancies per 100 women in the first year among non-breastfeeding women. Reported pregnancy rates in the first year of use range from 0% to 13%. Fertility returns immediately after being discontinued.

SAFETY AND ADVANTAGES

Progestin-only pills are safe as well as suitable for nearly all women, particularly for breastfeeding women who have resumed menstruation and want an oral contraceptive, although it is less effective than in fully breastfeeding women. POPs are safe even in breastfeeding women <6 months postpartum and breastfeeding woman before 6 weeks postpartum. They can be initiated immediately postabortion. POPs are a good option in whom estrogen is contraindicated or causes additional health concerns such as migraine with aura, >35 years of age, coronary artery disease, venous thromboembolic disease, and hypertension. POPs can be initiated without blood or other routine laboratory tests, pelvic examination, cervical cancer screening, or breast examination. They can be discontinued at any time without a provider's help. They are not going to interfere in sexual activity. There are no known health risks but *should not be given to women with current breast cancer or history of breast cancer.*

Progestin-only pills *protect against endometrial cancer* and against the reversible loss of bone density, which occurs in breastfeeding women. They do not cause significant weight gain.

DISADVANTAGES/SIDE EFFECTS

Progestin-only pills cause disruption of normal menstrual bleeding patterns—longer/delay in the return of monthly bleeding for breastfeeding women. One may have frequent, irregular, prolonged, or no monthly bleeding. POPs are associated with more functional ovarian cysts and acne flare than COCs.

MANAGING SIDE EFFECTS AND MISSING OF PILLS

Listen to client and give advice if required. Encourage to keep taking a tablet every day even if she has side effects as missing capsules can risk pregnancy. Explain that numerous side effects will subside after a month of use. For heavy bleeding, start tab tranexamic acid 500 mg 8 hourly. To prevent anemia, suggest taking iron tablets and taking foods containing iron similar as meat, egg, fish, green, lush vegetables, and legumes. If heavy or prolonged bleeding continues or starts after several months of normal or no yearly bleeding or if some other conditions, offer help to choose another system if she wishes or cannot overcome the problems.

CURRENT PROGESTIN-ONLY PILLS—DESOGESTREL

Desogestrel is a metabolite of etonogestrel, a potent progestin of the estrane steroid group, veritably picky, and has low androgenic action. Absorption takes place in the digestive tract and it gets converted to the active metabolite 3-keto-desogestrel. A 75 µg dose was preferred for clinical use as it showed the smallest degree of follicular development and the most respectable pattern of bleeding.[7] The 75 µg dose of desogestrel constantly inhibits ovulation without any advent androgenic goods and achieves a Pearl Index of 0.14, analogous to that of with COCs (0.05–0.4 according to studies). It has become an important and dependable option for all ages' women who wish to take oral contraception, whether breastfeeding or not, contraindicated for estrogens, those who do not want to gain weight, have dysmenorrhea, or want lower menstrual bleeding.[6] The POP containing desogestrel has higher contraceptive effectiveness than that of other POPs and in breastfeeding women, it is 100% higher than in non-breastfeeding women.[7]

Use of Desogestrel

Anovulation is considered to be done in 97% of cycles, without clinical benefits on lipids and carbohydrate metabolism and hemostasis.[8] There are no significant changes in systolic or diastolic blood pressure, weight gain, body mass index (BMI), or heart rate. There are salutary effects on hemostasis, without variations in antithrombin-III and protein C. Desogestrel does not increase the thrombotic or embolic venous threat.[8] Also observed is a significant reduction of factor-VII exertion, an independent threat for arterial complaint.[8] Decreased fibrinogen and plasminogen activator inhibitor-1 (PAI-I), which present a threat for arterial complaint when increased, noted by Schindler.[9]

Progestin-only pill containing desogestrel must be administered at the same time; because of the ovulation inhibitory effect, it is anticipated that a detention *of over to 12 hours does not affect contraceptive effectiveness* as the restoration of the hypothalamic-pituitary-ovarian axis takes further time.[10] The cooperative Study Group10 suggests the Pearl Index of desogestrel was 0.14 and that of levonorgestrel was 1.17, a major difference. Desogestrel has more pronounced repression of the hypothalamic-pituitary-ovarian axis with further inhibition of ovulation. In the cited study,[9] ectopic gestation was observed with levonorgestrel and not with desogestrel.

Noncontraceptive Benefits of Progestin-only Pills

Desogestrel can ameliorate dysmenorrhea. It can drop pain related to endometriosis and ameliorate premenstrual pressure.[11,12] It should be emphasized that over the period of time, use of the desogestrel POP shows reduction in the quantum and frequency of bleeding, amenorrhea becomes longer, and heavy/irregular bleeding tends to be less common.[11] The desogestrel POP is a timely oral contraceptive in circumstances where COCs should not be used,[13] even in breastfeeding.[14,15] POP containing desogestrel has a positive effect on the course of migraine in utmost women. POPs may be applicable for women over 35 years of age and may also help postpartum bone loss.[13]

FUTURE PROGESTIN-ONLY PILLS—DROSPIRENONE

Drospirenone derives from 17alpha-spironolactone, having parcels analogous to those of natural progesterone with bot antiandrogenic and antimineralocorticoid effects. Rosenbaum et al.[16] concluded inhibition of ovarian exertion and ovulation was cure dependent. Later, Duijkers et al.[17] evaluated 4.0 mg of drospirenone using the *24/4-day intake regimen (four days of a hormone-free interval as it has been used in COCs)*, showing effective ovarian repression. The permeability of cervical mucus was suppressed in both groups and the number of days of bleeding or finding was lower in the drospirenone group. POP containing drospirenone inhibited ovulation with the same efficacity as desogestrel, despite the 4-day interval without hormones. Archer et al.[18] published the results—the estimated global Pearl Index was 0.51 [95% confidence interval (CI) 0.1053–1.4922]. Unanticipated bleeding dropped from 49.1 in the first cycle to 22.8 at the end of the evaluation. Prolonged/heavy bleeding also dropped from 6.5 during cycles 2–4 to 4.2 during cycles 11–13. No evidence of deep vein thrombosis, hyperkalemia, pulmonary embolism or any significant changes in laboratory tests, body weight, body mass indicator, blood pressure, or heart rate were reported. Regidor et al.[19] set up due to its pharmacological parcels, it may be a valid volition to other POPs and indeed to COCs since it will not confer thromboembolic threat. The antiandrogenic and antimineralocorticoid effects, reduction of acne, and weight gain would eventually lead to a high position of adequacy and compliance.[20] In spite the 4-day hormone-free period, inhibition of ovulation was maintained. POP containing 4.0 mg of drospirenone in a 24/4-day intake regimen, unlike other POPs, it offers an important window of contraceptive effectiveness in spite of detainments or missed pills. All these studies have opened the doors for POP containing 4.0 mg of drospirenone in a 24/4-day intake regimen and contraceptive effectiveness analogous to that of COCs a good safety profile and more favorable cycle control than other POPs. Hadji, Colli, and Regidor concluded that progestin-only contraceptives do not appear to lead to an accelerated loss of bone mineral viscosity.[20] If the original results are verified in larger studies or in clinical practice, POP containing drospirenone will be one of the best contraceptive without estrogen, free of the topmost disadvantage of the other POPs The vacuity of this new POP that is effective, well-permitted, and with a predictable bleeding pattern, is veritably good news and has a promising place in contraception. It has begun to be promoted and used widely under the name of drospirenone-only pills (DOP). From a cardiovascular point of view, POPs are safer than COCs.[19] Will POP containing drospirenone in a 24/4-day intake regimen start the end of COC use? Only time, studies, and users will determine this. The WHO MEC should be applied before defining POP.

CONCLUSION

In hormonal contraception methods and birth control, POPs plays a major role. Over the period of time, they have come much further than minipills or pills for breastfeeding women. The vacuity of distinct progestins, without the presence of estrogen, can offer the same contraceptive efficacity offered by COCs, indeed while breastfeeding, is a sensitive advance. POPs containing levonorgestrel, other androgenic progestins, and desogestrel, as well as subdermal have been given continuously. In the third decade of the 21st century, POP containing drospirenone, administered by 24/4-day regimen with pause days, is available for the first time. Incorrectly, POPs are beginning to be available, offering the same contraceptive efficacity and analogous cycle control as COCs, without much adverse effects, pitfalls, and adverse impact on the integrity of the user, which are disadvantages of the use of contraceptives containing estrogen. "New" POPs with desogestrel or drospirenone should be favored over aged phrasings. POP with drospirenone may lead to the end of COCs if women's acceptance and menstrual cycle behavior are satisfied, as studies suggest. New progestins, or substances with progestin action, may be available in the future as birth control options acclimatized to women's comfort, demands, and satisfaction.

REFERENCES

1. OCHA. (2014). FP2020 Partnership in Progress 2013-2014. [online] Available from: https://reliefweb.int/report/world/fp2020-partnership-progress-2013-2014 [Last accessed January, 2024].
2. World Health Organization (WHO). Medical Eligibility Criteria for Contraceptive Use: A WHO Family Planning Cornerstone, 5th edition. Geneva: WHO; 2015.
3. Ministry of Health and Family Welfare Initiatives & Achievements-2023. New Delhi: PIB; 2015.
4. Latkin CA, Knowlton AR. Social network assessments and interventions for health behavior change: A critical review. Behav Med. 2015;41:90-7.
5. Grimes DA, Lopez LM, O'Brien PA, Raymond EG. Progestin-only pills for contraception. Cochrane Database Syst Rev. 2013;(11):CD007541.
6. World Health Organization (WHO) Department of Reproductive Health and Research, Johns Hopkins Bloomberg School of Public Health Center for Communication Programs (CCP) Knowledge for Health Project, United States Agency for International Development Bureau for Global Health Office of Population and Reproductive Health. (2011). Family Planning: A Global Handbook for Providers. [online] Available from: https://www.glowm.com/pdf/Family%20planning%20-%20a%20global%20handbook%20for%20providers.pdf [Last accessed January, 2024].
7. Collaborative Study Group on the Desogestrel containing progestogen only pill. A double blind study comparing the contraceptive efficacy, acceptability and safety of two progestogen only pills containing desogestrel 75 ug/day or Levonorgestrel 30 ug/day. Eur J Contracept Reprod Health Care. 1998;3(4):169-78.
8. Jeng CJ, Chuang L, Shen J. A comparison of progestogens or oral contraceptives and gonadotropin-releasing hormone agonists for the treatment of endometriosis: a systematic review. Expert Opin Pharmacother. 2014;15:767-7.
9. Schindler AE. Differential effects of progestins on hemostasis. Maturitas. 2003;46:31-7.
10. Korver T, Klipping C, Heger-Mahn D, Duijkers I, van Osta G, Dieben T. Maintenance of ovulation inhibition with the

75- μg desogestrel-only contraceptive pill (Cerazette®) after scheduled 12-hour delays in tablet intake. Contraception. 2005;71: 8-13.
11. Raymond E. Progestin-only pills. In: Hatcher RA, Trussell J, Nelson AL, Cates W, Kowal D, MS P (Eds). Contraceptive Technology, 20th edition. New York: Ardent Media; 2011. pp. 237-47.
12. Black A, Guilbert E. Canadian Contraceptive Consensus. Clinical practice guideline. J Obstet Gynaecol Can. 2016;38(3):279-300.
13. Costa ML, Cecatti JG, Krupa FG, Rehder PM, Sousa MH, Costa-Paiva L. Progestin-only contraception prevents bone loss in postpartum breastfeeding women. Contraception. 2012;85:374-80.
14. Le Moigne E, Tromeur C, Delluc A, Gouillou M, Alavi Z, Lacut K, et al. Risk of recurrent venous thromboembolism on progestin-only contraception: a cohort study. Haematologica. 2016;101(1):e12-4.
15. Nappi RE, Merki-Feld GS, Terreno E, Pellegrinelli A, Viana M. Hormonal contraception in women with migraine: is progestogen-only contraception a better choice? J Headache Pain. 2013;14(1):66.
16. Rosenbaum P, Schmidt W, Helmerhorst FM, Wuttke W, Rossmanith W, Freundl F, et al. Inhibition of ovulation by a novel progestogen drospirenone alone or in combination with ethinylestradiol. Eur J Contracept Reprod Health Care. 2000;5(1):16-24.
17. Duijkers IJ, Heger-Mahn D, Drouin D, Skouby S. A randomized study comparing the effect on ovarian activity of a progestogen-only pill (POP) containing desogestrel and a new POP containing drospirenone in a 24/4 regimen. Eur J Contracept Reprod Health Care. 2015;20(6):419-27.
18. Archer DF, Ahrendt HJ, Drouin D. Drospirenone-only oral contraceptive: results from a multicenter noncomparative trial of efficacy, safety and tolerability. Contraception. 2015;92(5):439-44.
19. Regidor PA, Colli E, Schindler AE. Drospirenone as estrogen-free pill and hemostasis: coagulatory study results comparing a novel 4 mg formulation in a 24 + 4 cycle with desogestrel 75 mg per day. Gynecol Endocrinol. 2016;32(9):749-51.
20. Hadji P, Colli E, Regidor PA. Bone health in estrogen-free contraception. Osteoporos Int. 2019;30(12):2391-400.

CHAPTER 4

Contraceptive Implants

Poonam Varma Shivkumar, Bhakthraj D Thombre

INTRODUCTION

Contraceptive implants are the latest method for the birth control. they are also known as LARCs (long-acting reversible contraceptives).

HISTORY

In 1966, scientist of population council began investigating the use of silicon rubber capsule as a way to continuously release steroid hormones and they concluded that this was possible with the effects form the hormones lasting a year or longer in animal models.[1] In 1975, a randomized controlled trial taking place in multiple centers across the six countries determined that the implants containing levonorgestrel were the best option in terms of safety and efficacy. In 1983, the NORPLANT came into the market. The World Health Organization evaluated and recommended the system worldwide as contraceptive device in 1984.[2] It was approved by the Food and Drug Administration (FDA) in 1990. In 2006, the FDA approved "Implanon", a single thin, plastic, levonorgestrel releasing rod. In 2010, Implanon was replaced by Nexplanon, which is designed to be radio-opaque and has an improved insertion device.[3]

DESCRIPTION

Contraceptive implants are the long-acting reversible contraceptives (LARCs), which were required once per cycle administration or even less. Implants consist of small rods of varying sizes made up of silicone, polyurethane, polyethylene, which releases hormones such as progesterone into the bloodstream in a long-period time which can extend up to 5 years. Contraceptive implants available in the market which are as follows:

- *LNG implants (levonorgestrel implants):* It consists of two implants and it is inserted with the help of disposable trocar. Two products available are "NORPLANT" and "NORPLANT-2 (Jadelle)".
- *Norplant:* This implant consists of six capsules each having 36 mg of LNG, total containing 216 mg of LNG. The capsule is 2.4 mm wide and 34 mm wide. It is approved for 5 years use.
- *Norplant-2 (Jadelle):* This implant consists of 2 LNG rods. Each rod contains 75 mg of LNG.
- Each rod has diameter of 2.5 mm and 43 mm in length. It is effective for 5 years.[4]
- *Etonogestrel implants*: It is single rod system, which is inserted with the help of special applicator.
- *Implanon/Nexplanon:* It is etonogestrel implants available in the market. It is a single-rod implant system. It measures about 2 mm in diameter and 4 cm in length. 68 mg of etonogestrel contains at the core of the implants; it is dispersed in a

matrix of ethylene-vinyl-acetate polymer. This implant contains 15 mg of barium sulfate ($BaSO_4$) which makes implants radiopaque.[5]

MECHANISM OF ACTION

Contraceptive implants prevent the sperm penetration in cervical mucus and the implantation by attenuating the endometrium and prevent the ovulation. The effectivity of the contraceptive implants is affected by the inducers such as antiretroviral therapy and antiepileptic drugs.[6]

INSERTION

Timing of Insertion

Implants are very effective when inserted during the first 5 days of the menstrual cycle. However, implants can be used anytime during the women's menstrual cycle. Implant is effective after 7 days of insertion. So, alternative contraception such as condom needs to be used for 7 days after installation to prevent unwanted pregnancy.[7]

For postpartum, insertion is performed after 21 days postpartum. Postabortion, insertion of the implant can be performed after 15 days of the abortion.

Technique of Insertion of Implant

It is a minor surgical procedure done under local anesthesia and performed by the trained provider on outpatient basis. Site of insertion is marked on upper inner aspect of the patient's nondominant arm 8–10 cm above the medial epicondyle and overlying the triceps muscle to avoid nerve and vessel injury. Implant should be inserted subdermally. Applicator should be held with 30° slope to the skin and thereafter immediately after the needle penetrates the dermis is lowered to the horizontal position.[8]

Advantages of Implants

- It is effective after a few hours of insertion.
- Fertility returns within 3–4 weeks of removal and ovulation rate is >90% after removal of implant.
- Implants contain only progesterone, so there is not any estrogenic side effect.
- It decreases blood flow during menses, so decreases incidence of anemia.
- Low risk of ectopic pregnancy
- Pregnancy rate is 0.2–0.5 per 100 women per year.
- It does not interfere with breastfeeding.

Contraindication for Implant use

- Recent thromboembolic disorder or past history of thrombosis
- Active liver disease or carcinoma of liver
- Undiagnosed abnormal genital tumor
- Known case or suspected breast cancer
- Allergic reaction to implants
- Known or suspected pregnancy.

Side Effect of Implants

Local: It includes pain, redness, or irritation over the insertion site.

Systemic:

- *Menstrual abnormalities:* Most common side effect of implants is irregular, uterine bleeding which occur in almost 11% of the users. It is associated with longer or shorter duration of menstrual cycles, or amenorrhea.[9]
- *Risk of sexually acquired infection:* Implants do not protect against sexually transmitted infections. Women with multiple sexual partners should be counseled regarding concomitant condom use to provide protection against sexually transmitted infection.
- *Other side effects:* It includes headache (16%), weight gain (12%), acne (12%),

breast tenderness (10%), emotional liabilities (6%), and abdominal pain (5%).
- *Timing of removal:* Implants can be removed at any time, but it should be removed after 3 or 5 years of the insertion. After removal of implants circulating levels of etonogestrel became undetectable in 1 week. After removal of implants ovulation occur in 3–4 weeks in 90% of the patient.[10]

SUMMARY

Contraceptive implants are long-acting reversible contraceptives (LARCs) with progesterone as the main hormone. It is free from the estrogenic side effects so this can be used safely in patients in whom estrogen-containing contraceptives contraindicated. It can be used in breastfeeding women earlier as compared to the estrogen-containing contraceptives.[11] It is used safely among the sexually active adolescents. It does not provide any protection against sexually transmitted infections.

REFERENCES

1. Power J, French R, Cowan FM. Subdermal implantable contraceptives versus other forms of reversible contraceptives or other implants as effective methods for preventing pregnancy. Cochrane Database Syst Rev. 2007;2007(3):CD001326.
2. Ramchandran D, Upadhyay UD. Implants: the next generation. Popul Reports Ser K Inject Implant; 2007;1-19.
3. Jacobstein R, Polis CB. Progestin-only contraception: injectables and implants. Best Pract Res Clin Obstet Gynaecol. 2014;28: 795-806.
4. Reproductive Health Supplies Coalition. Caucus on New and Underused Reproductive Health Technologies. Cochrane Database Syst Rev. 2011;12-4.
5. Faculty of Sexual and Reproductive Healthcare. Clinical Guidance: Drug Interactions with Hormonal Contraception Drug Interactions with Hormonal Contraception; 2017. pp. 1-12.
6. Faculty of Sexual and Reproductive Healthcare. Introduction: Effectiveness of Contraceptive Method. UK Med Eligibility Criteria Contracept. UK: Faculty of Sexual and Reproductive Healthcare; 2016. pp. 1-7.
7. Stoddard A, McNicholas C, Peipert JF. Efficacy and safety of long-acting reversible contraception. Drugs. 2011;71:969-80.
8. Russo JA, Miller E, Gold MA. Myths and misconceptions about long-acting reversible contraception (LARC). J Adolesc Health. 2013;52:S14-21.
9. US Food and Drug Administration (FDA) approved product information. (2021). Nexplanon-etonogestrel implant. Revised July, 2021. US National Library of Medicine. [online] Available from: https://dailymed.nlm.nih.gov/dailymed/drugInfo.cfm?setid=b03a3917-9a65-45c2-bbbb-871da858ef34 [Last accessed December, 2022].
10. Darney P, Patel A, Rosen K, Shapiro LS, Kaunitz AM. Safety and efficacy of a single-rod etonogestrel implant (Implanon): Results from 11 international clinical trials. Fertil Steril. 2009;91:1646-53.
11. Mansour HM, Sohn MJ, Al-Ghananeem A, DeLuca PP. Materials for pharmaceutical dosage forms: molecular pharmaceutics and controlled release drug delivery aspects. Int J Mol Sci. 2010;11:3298-322.

CHAPTER 5

Contraceptive Vaginal Ring

Ruchika Garg, Malavika JC

CONTRACEPTIVE VAGINAL RING

Contraceptive vaginal ring is a form of combined hormonal contraceptive method. Combined (estrogen-progestin) hormonal contraception is available in various forms such as an oral pill, transdermal patch or a vaginal ring. All these methods are user-controlled. When used consistently and correctly, they are safe and highly effective.

What is a vaginal ring?

Contraceptive vaginal ring is a small flexible soft plastic ring that is placed inside the vagina. It releases both estrogen and progesterone continuously into the bloodstream, thereby preventing pregnancy. The main advantage of vaginal ring over other combined methods is the *longer duration of action* and avoids the difficulty with daily or weekly use and hence ensures *better compliance.*

What are the types of vaginal ring available in the market?

Combined hormonal contraceptive vaginal rings are available under the following brand names:

NuvaRing: It is a 1-month ring. It is flexible latex-free device measuring around 2 inches in diameter. It contains ethinyl estradiol (EE) and etonogestrel (ENG). It needs to be worn in the vagina for 3 weeks and removed and discarded for 1 week. It releases 120 µg of EE and 15 µg of ENG continuously into the bloodstream over 21 days.[1] The dose of EE released by the vaginal ring is much lower than that released by other combined hormonal contraceptive methods.

Annovera: It is a 1-year ring. It can be rinsed and reinserted every month. Overall it can be used for 13 cycles. It contains EE and segesterone acetate (SA). The ring has to be placed in the vagina for 3 weeks and removed for 1 week. Annovera comes with a case to safely store the ring during the ring free week.[2]

MECHANISM OF ACTION

Both estrogen and progesterone are continuously released into the bloodstream.

Estrogen acts by preventing ovulation and progesterone acts by thickening the cervical mucus making it difficult for the sperm to enter the cervix and even the endometrium is rendered hostile for implantation.

Time to Insert the Vaginal Ring

Vaginal ring can be inserted at any time of the menstrual cycle provided pregnancy is ruled out.

If the vaginal ring is inserted in the vagina within first 5 days of menstrual cycle, then the chances of pregnancy is very less.

If the vaginal ring is inserted in any other time of the menstrual cycle then additional contraception needs to be used for first 7 days after insertion to avoid pregnancy.

Ideally, ring should be left in the vagina for 21 days and removed for 7 days. There is protection against pregnancy in the ring-free period. There is also a choice for the woman to have a shorter ring-free break or no break at all. This is known to be as safe and effective as the standard use (7-day break).

The partner may feel the vaginal ring while having sex but it is not harmful.

Postpartum Insertion

vaginal ring can be used safely by breast-feeding woman after 42 days of giving birth, a back-up contraception should be used for 7 days in such situations.

If the woman is not breast-feeding and vaginal ring is inserted on day 21 after giving birth, then no back-up contraception is needed. If it is >21 of days of giving birth, then additional contraception should be used for first 7 days of the ring insertion.

Postabortion insertion: Vaginal ring can be inserted immediately after abortion without the need of back-up contraception.

If 5 days has elapsed since abortion, then a back-up contraception needs to be used for 7 days after the insertion of the ring.

How to insert the vaginal ring?

After cleaning the hands, the ring needs to be squeezed between the thumb and the finger and should be gently inserted into the vagina and the ring should be pushed up till it feels comfortable. It is not required for the ring to completely cover the cervix as with diaphragm and cervical cap.

After the ring is inside the vagina for 21 days (3 weeks), then it should be removed. After a ring free period of 7 days a new ring should be inserted .

The ring should be inserted on the same day of the week when it was removed. For example, if the ring was removed on Monday, then a new ring should be inserted the next Monday and the ring should be removed after 3 weeks on Monday itself.

Delayed Insertion

- Woman who forget to insert a new ring on time and if it is <48 hours due for insertion of a new ring, then the woman can insert the ring immediately without the need for additional contraception.[3]
- If the woman has forgotten to insert the new ring for >48 hours, then a new ring should be inserted immediately and an additional contraception is needed for 7 days.

How to remove the vaginal ring?

With clean hands, insert a finger into the vagina, hook around its edge and gently pull out the ring. After removing the ring, it should be placed in a bag provided and thrown into the bin. There should not be any pain while removing the ring. In case of Annovera, the ring should be rinsed, cleaned, and placed in a case.

In the ring-free interval, there can be a period type bleed.

After 7 days ring-free period, insert a new vaginal ring. The new ring can be placed irrespective of the menstrual bleed.

DELAYED REMOVAL

If the NuvaRing is in situ for >3 weeks but <5 weeks, then remove the ring and insert a new ring after 1-week ring-free period. If the woman desires, she can insert a new ring immediately after removing the old one fore-going the 1-week ring-free interval, although the woman may experience breakthrough bleeding.

If the NuvaRing is in situ for >5 weeks then the ring should be removed and replaced with a new ring immediately. But, an additional contraception like condoms is necessary for the first 7 days following insertion of the new vaginal ring.

Rationale behind this is the fact that sufficient amount of estrogen and progesterone is released by the vaginal ring to prevent pregnancy (by inhibition of ovulation) for 5 weeks. Hence, even if the woman forgets removing the vaginal ring after 3 weeks, the efficacy is maintained up to 5 weeks.[4]

What if the vaginal ring falls out?

For NuvaRing: If the ring falls out, then the ring should be cleaned and placed in the vagina immediately.

If the ring has been out of the vagina for >3 hours, then a back-up contraception should be used.

For Annovera: If the ring falls out or it is out of the vagina for up to 2 hours, then the ring is washed with a mild soap and water and dried and inserted into the vagina and no back up contraception needed.[2]

If the ring is out of the vagina for >2 hours, then re-insert the ring after washing it, and an additional contraception (e.g., condoms) is needed for 7 days.

How to take care of the vaginal ring?

Place NuvaRing at room temperature. It should be kept away from direct sunlight. In such conditions, it can be stored up to 4 months.

If the NuvaRing is not used within 4 months, then it has to be stored in the refrigerator.

Annovera, once removed out of the vagina should be washed with a mild soap and lukewarm water, dried with a clean cloth or a paper towel and stored in a case. Avoid extreme temperatures.

Annovera, when placed inside the vagina, concurrent use of oil or silicone-based products like suppositories, creams, gels, and lubricants should be avoided. Water-based lubricants can be used.

ADMINISTRATION AND USE

Before Prescribing Vaginal Ring

- Pregnancy should be excluded.
- *Measure blood pressure*: Ideally, blood pressure should be measured before starting any form of combined hormonal contraceptives.
- Physical examination and laboratory tests are not mandatory.[3]

Who can use the vaginal ring?

Woman without the following conditions may use the vaginal ring.

Vaginal ring is not suitable for women with:
- History of arterial or venous thrombosis
- Hypertensive and cardiac problems
- Age >35 years
- Overweight
- Smoking or stopped smoking recently in the past 1 year
- History of migraine with aura (warning symptoms)
- Suffering from breast cancer or had breast cancer in the past 5 years.
- Diabetic with complications
- Taking medicines which interact with the ring
- Cannot hold the ring in the vagina.

If the woman does not smoke and is not suffering from any medical comorbidities then the vaginal ring can be used in woman up to 50 years of age.

BENEFITS AND RISKS OF VAGINAL RING

Benefits

- It does not interfere with sex.
- Improved compliance as the woman does not have to think about it every day.
- It is easy insert and remove.
- Action of vaginal ring is unaffected by conditions like vomiting and diarrhea.

- Provides better cycle control and reduces bleeding and dysmenorrhea.
- It helps woman with premenstrual symptoms.

Risks

- At the beginning, woman may not feel comfortable inserting and removing the vaginal ring.
- Vaginal ring does not protect against sexually transmitted infections.
- Interaction with some drugs may render it less effective.
- Woman needs to remember the day on which vaginal ring needs to be removed and when the new one needs to be inserted.
- Sometimes the ring can get expelled during the act of sex or following a bowel movement.
- Some woman may experience spotting and bleeding in the first few months following insertion.
- It may cause increased vaginal discharge.
- Headaches, nausea, breast tenderness, and mood changes can occur just as with other combined hormonal methods.

Serious Risks

Vaginal rings carry same serious risk as with any other combined hormonal methods.

Cardiovascular and thromboembolic events—combined hormonal contraceptives are known to increase the risk of thromboembolic events compared to the nonusers.[1,2] Although the risk of VTE is lower in ring users compared to other combined methods.[5]

Hence, woman with a history of previous VTE should not choose a vaginal ring.

Risk of Cancer

Women using vaginal ring have a very small increased risk of being diagnosed with breast cancer but this risk reduces once the woman stops using the ring.

There is also a small increased risk of developing cervical cancer with long-term use of any combined hormonal contraception.

FOLLOW-UP

- A routine follow-up examination is not needed.
- Blood pressure should be checked yearly.

RETURN OF FERTILITY

Majority of woman resume ovulation and regular menses within a month of removal of vaginal rings.[1] In a study conducted on 45 participants using NuvaRing, ovulation was reported to be as early as 13 days after removal of ring and the median time to ovulate was 19 days after removal of vaginal ring.[6] Similarly, with Annovera initial trials reported return of regular menses within 6 months of discontinuation.[2]

Use with Other Vaginal Devices and Products

Vaginal rings are known to interfere with other female barrier contraceptive methods such as diaphragm, cervical cap, or the female condoms. Hence, female barrier contraceptives cannot be used as back-up contraception along with vaginal rings.[7]

Concomitant use of tampons during menses does not affect the hormone absorption from the vaginal ring.[1]

Vaginal rings are compatible with water-based vaginal lubricants and spermicides, but oil-based products including silicone-based lubricants are not compatible with vaginal rings.[1,2]

INTERACTIONS WITH OTHER MEDICATIONS

Interactions of vaginal ring is similar to COCs and most of the information is based on it.

Vaginal rings interact with other systemic medications and consequently increase or decrease each other's levels.

- *Decrease in estrogen/progestin levels:* Drugs which increase the activity of liver microsomal enzymes decrease systemic exposure to the estrogen and progestins in contraceptive vaginal rings, and thus contraceptive efficacy is reduced.

Some such medications are:

- Antiepileptics such as barbiturate, phenytoin, carbamazepine, oxcarbazepine, and topiramate.
- Antifungal like griseofulvin.
- Antitubercular drugs such as rifampicin and rifabutin.
- Anti-HIV medications such as efavirenz, nelfinavir, ritonavir, darunavir, lopinavir, and nevirapine.[1,2]
- Individuals using the above medications should use an additional form of contraception such as condoms or choose an alternative form of contraceptions.

Altered Levels of Certain Medications

Plasma levels of lamotrigine is known to decrease when used along with combined hormonal methods. Hence, seizure control may not be optimal and a higher dose of lamotrigine may be needed to attain good seizure control.[8,9]

Combined hormonal methods are avoided in those women on antiviral medications for hepatitis C (ritonavir and paritaprevir) since ALT levels are significantly elevated.

Use with other vaginal medications: Water-based vaginal drugs used in treatment of vaginal candidiasis or bacterial vaginosis can be used along with vaginal rings.[1,2]

Oil-based suppositories such as miconazole suppositories are associated with increased hormonal levels and hence avoided along with vaginal rings.[1,2]

SPECIAL SITUATIONS

- If the vaginal ring is out for unknown duration of time, then pregnancy has to be ruled out before inserting a new ring.[7]
- *Continuous use of ring for menstrual suppression*: Some women desire fewer days of withdrawal bleed and may prefer using vaginal ring for extended period. Vaginal ring may be used without ring-free period wherein a new ring is inserted immediately after the removal of old ring. This omits hormone-free interval. Extended use of ring is effective but the woman may suffer from unscheduled bleeding and spotting.[10,11]
- Data supporting continuous use of the Annovera are not yet available, but continuous use may be associated with increase in unscheduled bleeding.
- *Broken ring*—very rarely, the contraceptive ring may break at the weld joint.[1] The break does not affect the contraceptive effectiveness, but it is more likely that the ring slips out. Hence in the event of broken ring, the ring needs to be removed and replaced with a new one.

NONCONTRACEPTIVE BENEFITS OF VAGINAL RING

Cycle control: Cycle control is a major benefit provided by all combined hormonal contraceptive methods. In this regard, vaginal ring is equivalent or possibly superior to other combined hormonal contraceptives.[12-14]

Vaginal ring users less frequently experience breakthrough bleeding unlike with other combined methods.[12,14-16]

Endometriosis: Vaginal ring appears to reduce endometriosis-related pain. A cohort study was conducted comparing NuvaRing with a transdermal patch for relief of persistent endometriosis-related pain and it was reported that both treatments reduced dysmenorrhea,[13] but ring users were more satisfied compared to the patch users (72 vs. 48%).

Diabetic or prediabetic woman: Woman who are diagnosed with insulin resistance or those who are at risk of insulin resistance may benefit from the contraceptive ring as compared to COCs because the vaginal ring had no impact on insulin resistance while COCs were known to increase insulin levels.[17]

Improved psychosexual function: Vaginal ring users have been studied to have improved psychosexual function.[18-20]

What is correct use?

Correct and consistent use of the contraceptive vaginal ring is very similar to other combined hormonal methods.

NuvaRing should be ideally placed used as three weeks in and 1 week out. Some women prefer to extend the use for up to 5 weeks to regulate their cycles.[15,21,22]

When used correctly, the ring is almost 99% effective in preventing pregnancy.

The Centers for Disease Control and Prevention (CDC) reports a 7% pregnancy rate with typical use.

ACCEPTABILITY OF VAGINAL RINGS

Vaginal rings are highly acceptable as it is easy to use, once a month administration, remains effective even if removal or reinsertion of the ring is not done precisely on time.

A low level of systemic hormone is maintained enough to prevent ovulation (vaginal delivery of hormones improve its bioavailability).

Even the effect is rapidly reversible. Users of NuvaRing report a satisfaction rates of 84–96% and are more likely to recommend the method to other women.[21,23,24]

Minor complaints like feeling of the ring, coital problems, and expulsion of the ring are complained by <3% of the women.[25,26]

Compared to COCs vaginal ring users are more satisfied.[25,26]

Vaginal ring users are less likely to discontinue as compared to COC users (11% vs. 16%).

SUMMARY: FACTS ABOUT THE VAGINAL RING

When used correctly and consistently:

- Vaginal ring is >99% effective.
- Compliance is better since each ring provides contraception for a month.
- Does not interfere with sex when the ring is in place.
- Vaginal rings do not protect against STI, and hence condoms may be used concomitantly.
- Unlike COCs, vaginal ring works even when the woman has vomiting or diarrhea.
- Regular menses is lighter, less painful, and also prevents premenstrual symptoms.
- Minimal side effects like white discharge may be there.
- Complications like VTEs are rare but a possibility.
- When the ring comes out accidentally, it should be washed with mild soap and water and dried and re-inserted in the vagina.
- *To improve the effectiveness, a new ring should be inserted on the same day of the week when it was removed.*

TABLE 1: Comparison of vaginal ring to other birth control methods.

	Ring	***Patch***	***Pill***	***Shot***	***IUD***	***Implant***
Effectiveness (typical use)	93%	93%	93%	96%	• 99.2% (Copper) • 99.6% (Hormonal)	99.9%
Schedule	Replace monthly	Replace weekly	Take daily	Get every 3 months	Lasts up to 12 years	Lasts up to 5 years
Risks	Rare, but include: • Blood clots • Stroke • Heart attack	Rare, but include: • Blood clots • Stroke • Heart attack	Rare, but include: • Heart attack • Blood clots • Stroke • Liver tumors	Temporary osteoporosis	• Loss of the IUD or IUD moving out of place • Ectopic pregnancy • Infection	• Scarring • Infection
Side effects	• Sore breasts • Spotting • Headaches • Nausea	• Sore breasts • Spotting • Headaches • Nausea	• Sore breasts • Spotting • Headaches • Nausea	• Changes to your period • Nausea • Weight gain • Headaches • Depression • Sore breasts • bruising at the injection site	• Pain during insertion and days afterward • Irregular periods and spotting for hormonal IUD • More bleeding and cramping during periods for copper IUD	• Arm pain • Heavier, longer periods in some people • Headaches • Weight gain • Ovarian cysts • Nausea • Breast pain

- When the ring is out of the vagina for >3 hours, then an additional back-up contraception should be used.
- When medications interacting with the vaginal ring is taken, an additional back-up contraception is advised.

RECENT DEVELOPMENTS IN VAGINAL RINGS

- *Progering*: A new progesterone releasing vaginal ring widely available in South America and Africa, commonly advised for lactating woman.[27,28]

  Each ring releases 10 mg progesterone daily. It is approved for 3 months use. It acts to thicken the cervical mucus and also inhibits ovulation and affects endometrial receptivity. Unscheduled bleeding is a common complaint.[29] A ring that releases a synthetic progestin (Nesterone) is under development.
- A newer combined hormonal ring containing estrogen in the form of EE and progesterone in the form of Nesterone, a 19-nortestosterone derivative is under trial. Nestrone does not bind to either estrogen or androgen receptors and hence side effects like acne are reduced. This novel method was created with the goal to reduce the thrombogenic risk.[30,31]

How does the vaginal ring compare to other birth control methods?
See **Table 1**.

REFERENCES

1. Nuvaring [package insert]. (2018). Whitehouse Station, NJ. Merck and Co, Inc. 2001-2018. [online] Available from: http://www.merck.com/product/usa/pi_circulars/n/nuvaring/nuvaring_pi.pdf. [Last accessed November, 2022].
2. Annovera [package insert]. New York, NY. Manufactured for Population Council. August 2018. [online] Available from www.accessdata.fda.gov/drugsatfda_docs/label/2018/209627s000lbl.pdf [Last accessed November, 2022].
3. Curtis KM, Jatlaoui TC, Tepper NK, et al. U.S. Selected Practice Recommendations for Contraceptive Use, 2016. MMWR Recomm Rep. 2016;65:1.
4. Mulders TM, Dieben TO. Use of the novel combined contraceptive vaginal ring NuvaRing for ovulation inhibition. Fertil Steril. 2001;75:865.
5. Han L, Jensen JT. Does the progestogen used in combined hormonal contraception affect venous thrombosis risk? Obstet Gynecol Clin North Am 2015;42:683.
6. Mulders TM, Dieben TO, Bennink HJ. Ovarian function with a novel combined contraceptive vaginal ring. Hum Reprod. 2002;17:2594.
7. Nuvaring-etonogestrel and ethinyl estradiol insert, extended release. US Food and Drug Administration (FDA) approved product information. Revised May 30, 2017. [online] Available from https://dailymed.nlm.nih.gov/dailymed/lookup.cfm?setid=1347d58b-c505-45e7-aa9d-9800b9cf40c5 [Last accessed November, 2022].
8. Curtis KM, Tepper NK, Jatlaoui TC. U.S. Medical Eligibility Criteria for Contraceptive Use, 2016. MMWR Recomm Rep. 2016;65:1.
9. Dragoman M, Curtis KM, Gaffield ME. Combined hormonal contraceptive use among women with known dyslipidemias: a systematic review of critical safety outcomes. Contraception. 2016;94:280.
10. Miller L, Verhoeven CH, Hout Ji. Extended regimens of the contraceptive vaginal ring: a randomized trial. Obstet Gynecol. 2005;106:473.
11. Barreiros FA, Guazzelli CA, Barbosa R, de Assis F, de Araújo FF. Extended regimens of the contraceptive vaginal ring: evaluation of clinical aspects. Contraception. 2010;81:223.
12. Bjarnadóttir RI, Tuppurainen M, Killick SR. Comparison of cycle control with a combined contraceptive vaginal ring and oral levonorgestrel/ethinyl estradiol. Am J Obstet Gynecol. 2002;186:389.
13. Vercellini P, Barbara G, Somigliana E, Bianchi S, Abbiati A, Fedele L. Comparison

of contraceptive ring and patch for the treatment of symptomatic endometriosis. Fertil Steril 2010;93:2150-61.
14. Westhoff C, Osborne LM, Schafer JE, Morroni C. Bleeding patterns after immediate initiation of an oral compared with a vaginal hormonal contraceptive. Obstet Gynecol. 2005;106:89.
15. Oddsson K, Leifels-Fischer B, de Melo NR, Wiel-Masson D, Benedetto C, Verhoeven CH, et al. Efficacy and safety of a contraceptive vaginal ring (NuvaRing) compared with a combined oral contraceptive: a 1-year randomized trial. Contraception. 2005;71:176-82.
16. Oddsson K, Leifels-Fischer B, Wiel-Masson D, de Melo NR, Benedetto C, Verhoeven CH, et al. Superior cycle control with a contraceptive vaginal ring compared with an oral contraceptive containing 30 microg ethinylestradiol and 150 microg levonorgestrel: a randomized trial. Hum Reprod. 2005;20:557-62.
17. Cagnacci A, Ferrari S, Tirelli A, , Zanin R, Volpe A. Route of administration of contraceptives containing desogestrel/etonorgestrel and insulin sensitivity: a prospective randomized study. Contraception. 2009;80:34-9.
18. Guida M, Di Spiezio Sardo A, Bramante S, Bramante S, Sparice S, Acunzo G, et al. Effects of two types of hormonal contraception—oral versus intravaginal—on the sexual life of women and their partners. Hum Reprod. 2005;20:1100-6.
19. Morotti E, Casadio P, Guasina F, Battaglia B, Mattioli M, Battaglia C. Weight gain, body image and sexual function in young patients treated with contraceptive vaginal ring. A prospective pilot study. Gynecol Endocrinol. 2017; 33:660-4.
20. Guida M, Cibarelli F, Troisi J, Gallo A, Palumbo AR, Di Spiezio Sardo A. Sexual life impact evaluation of different hormonal contraceptives on the basis of their methods of administration. Arch Gynecol Obstet. 2014;290:1239-47.
21. Roumen FJ, Apter D, Mulders TM, Dieben TO. Efficacy, tolerability and acceptability of a novel contraceptive vaginal ring releasing etonogestrel and ethinyl oestradiol. Hum Reprod. 2001;16:469.
22. Roumen FJ, op ten Berg MM, Hoomans EH. The combined contraceptive vaginal ring (NuvaRing): first experience in daily clinical practice in The Netherlands. Eur J Contracept Reprod Health Care 2006;11:14.
23. Dieben TO, Roumen FJ, Apter D. Efficacy, cycle control, and user acceptability of a novel combined contraceptive vaginal ring. Obstet Gynecol 2002;100:585.
24. Merki-Feld GS, Hund M. Clinical experience with NuvaRing in daily practice in Switzerland: cycle control and acceptability among women of all reproductive ages. Eur J Contracept Reprod Health Care. 2007;12:240.
25. Ahrendt HJ, Nisand I, Bastianelli C. Efficacy, acceptability and tolerability of the combined contraceptive ring, NuvaRing, compared with an oral contraceptive containing 30 microg of ethinyl estradiol and 3 mg of drospirenone. Contraception. 2006;74:451.
26. Schafer JE, Osborne LM, Davis AR, Westhoff C. Acceptability and satisfaction using Quick Start with the contraceptive vaginal ring versus an oral contraceptive. Contraception 2006;73:488.
27. RamaRao S, Obare F, Ishaku S, Mané B, Clark H, Liambila W, et al. Do Women Find the Progesterone Vaginal Ring Acceptable? Findings from Kenya, Nigeria, and Senegal. Stud Fam Plann 2018;49:71-86.
28. Massai R, Quinteros E, Reyes MV. Extended use of a progesterone-releasing vaginal ring in nursing women: a phase II clinical trial. Contraception. 2005;72:352.
29. Nath A, Sitruk-Ware R. Progesterone vaginal ring for contraceptive use during lactation. Contraception. 2010;82:428.
30. Jensen JT, Edelman AB, Chen BA, Archer DF, Barnhart KT, Thomas MA, et al. Continuous dosing of a novel contraceptive vaginal ring releasing Nestorone® and estradiol: pharmacokinetics from a dose-finding study. Contraception. 2018; 97:422-7.
31. Archer DF, Thomas MA, Conard J, Merkatz RB, Creasy GW, Roberts K, et al. Impact on hepatic estrogen-sensitive proteins by a 1-year contraceptive vaginal ring delivering Nestorone® and ethinyl estradiol. Contraception. 2016;93:58-64.

CHAPTER 6

Contraceptive Patches

Ashish Kale, Ashwini Kale

INTRODUCTION

Hormonal contraceptives are effective because they utilize an estrogen and progestin analog to avert pregnancies. Negative feedback at the hypothalamus mediates the contraceptive effect, leading to lower levels of follicle-stimulating hormone (FSH) and luteinizing hormone (LH) production from the pituitary gland. Ovulation cannot occur in the absence of the LH surge. Progestin also reduces the likelihood of implantation because it thickens cervical mucus, slows tubal motility, and prevents endometrial development.[1] This is the basic mechanism and hormones involved in all forms of the hormonal contraceptive delivery system but differing when comes to efficacy and safety related to their delivery methods thus affecting their usage.

Of all the forms of contraception that exist, contraceptive patches are one of the most common contraceptive methods used after oral contraception. The contraceptive patch **(Fig. 1)** is a drug-containing patch that is 5 cm^2 in area and is effective for a period of 7 days. It is a transdermal contraceptive patch that has a relatively short duration of action and is reversible. It delivers sustained low amounts of estrogen and progestin into the body.[2]

CONCEPTION OF AN AUTONOMY: THE CONTRACEPTIVE PATCHES

In the 1980s, the ethinyl estradiol (EE)/norelgestromin patch was the initial transdermal birth control patch to receive global approval and recognition. In a transdermal route, the molecule of the drug must be small and lipophilic to penetrate through the skin membrane easily. Estradiol and EE are ideal molecules at therapeutic levels and can be delivered easily, but progesterone and progestin require higher therapeutic levels to be effective.[3]

Each patch is designed to give a mix of EE and norelgestromin to the body for a period of 1 week. The patch is applied topically to healthy skin. Clinical equivalence to oral

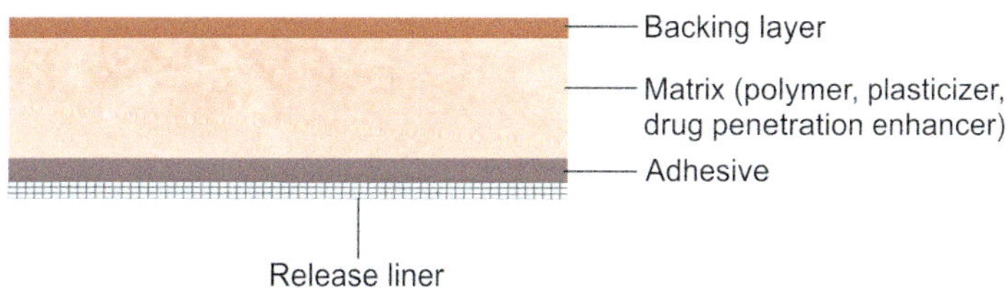

Fig. 1: Three-layered contraceptive patches.

contraceptives has been demonstrated for a treatment plan of 3 weeks with a patch on and 1 week without a patch for each menstrual cycle using the EE/norelgestromin patch.

BENEFITS OF TRANSDERMAL PATCH

Whatever may be the method of contraception, imperfect use of the method significantly increases the chances of pregnancy. One of the most common imperfections is adherence to a daily dose regimen especially when it is not an ailment. This issue can be improved by reducing the daily dosing schedule. A transdermal patch is a hormonal contraceptive that has currently achieved this goal.

Benefits in a nutshell:[4]

- Transdermal contraceptive patches are an efficient and convenient way of hormonal contraception.
- It is 99% effective in the prevention of pregnancy if used correctly.
- Women who desire a weekly application that does not involve daily oral contraceptions (OCs) will find it convenient.
- Eliminates the spikes and valleys in serum concentrations that are typical of OCs by acting as a buffer.
- It has a better rate of compliance and a lower rate of failure overall.
- The effectiveness of this method is comparable to that of oral and transvaginal contraception.
- It provides a dual benefit by giving relief during painful menstruation.
- Beneficial for women who are suffering from gastrointestinal problems.

SUPPORTING RESEARCH STUDIES

- When compared to pill users, the higher rates of correct and consistent use reported by patch users provided a better pregnancy protection potential in clinical trials **(Table 1)**.

TABLE 1: Percentage of cycles for which women (North American) reported correct and consistent method utilization, by age group.

	Correct and consistent use for 13 cycles (%)		
Age group (years)	***Transdermal patch***	***Oral contra-ceptive***	***Difference***
<20	87.8	67.7	20.1
20–24	88.3	74.4	13.9
25–29	88.3	79.8	8.5
30–34	89.4	85.2	4.2
35–39	88.3	82.6	5.7
>40	91.6	84.6	7.0
Overall	88.7	79.2	9.5

As can be seen in the table above, the proportion of cycles in which the patch was used correctly was significantly higher than the proportion of cycles in which women took their pills as advised (79.2% vs. 88.7%).

In the age group of 18–19 years old, the discrepancy between accurate patch use and pill use was greatest. While only 67.7% of pill users reported taking a pill daily for 13 cycles, accurate patch use was reported by 87.7% of users.[5]

- A Cochrane systematic review evaluated the effectiveness, cycle control, compliance, and safety of the contraceptive patch versus combination oral contraceptives. Self-reported adherence was higher with the patch, but overall efficacy was the same for both techniques.[6]
- In a trial conducted by Rubinstein et al. that comprised a small group of 50 teenagers, and a time period of 3 months, reported results as 77% of those who expected to continue using patches finished all

3 months (62% completed; 87.1% of completers confirmed flawless use).[7]

- In a retrospective trial of 62 teens performed by Logsdon et al. for 10 months, only 10 teenagers (16.7%) discontinued patch use; mostly due to economic causes.[8]
- In a separate trial, teenage girls who had used the patch for at least 6 months were questioned by Harel et al. All the women reported regular menses while using the patch; 93% claimed they had always remembered to apply a new patch on time and would recommend the patch to a friend.[9]
- A study performed by Archer DF et al., on 1,785 patch users showed a perfect use ranging from 88.1 to 91.0% across different age groups, implying good compliance among adolescent and adult users.[10]
- In a separate study, researchers found larger discrepancies between the age groups. This study encourages the method of contraceptive patch use which was significantly better when compared with an oral contraceptive. Moreover, the contraceptive patch is uniformly easy to use across all ages.[11]

POSSIBLE DISADVANTAGES OF TRANSDERMAL PATCH[12,13]

- Patches are contraindicated in active skin conditions, which could alter the rate of hormonal absorption or those dermatologic conditions that would worsen or flare up by patch application.
- Women with a body mass index >90 kg may be at a greater risk for pregnancy than women with a lower BMI.
- The patch can raise blood pressure, cause headaches and blood clots (rarely).
- May not be suitable for smokers.
- Like all other contraceptives, it does not provide safety from sexually transmitted diseases (STDs).

SIDE EFFECTS OF CONTRACEPTIVE PATCH

For first-time users, the side effects are mostly estrogens-related and are mild-to-moderate in severity. Among these symptoms include nausea, breast discomfort, emotional lability, and dysmenorrhea.

One exceptional adverse effect is application site reaction, which occurs on an average of 20% of users and limits usage in 2% of users.[14]

CONFLICTING ISSUE

A hugely undermined beneficial use of the transdermal patch is that the levels of estrogens are steady without the peaks and troughs that are seen with OC pills. This is because this advantage is accompanied by the area under curve (AUC) of estrogen being 60% higher in patch users even with a 35-µg dosage. In comparison to women who take pills, those who utilize patches have a higher overall estrogen exposure, which has led to major concerns and an increased risk of venous thromboembolism (VTE). Here, the facts get complicated.

Even though there is a discrepancy in the research, there is evidence to suggest that the patch increases the risk of a nonfatal thromboembolic event by a factor of two compared to OCs. The absolute risk of VTE is still quite low, even though the relative risk is relatively larger.

This is owing to the fact that the degree to which a method influences the generation of clotting factors is directly proportional to the amount of estrogen that is delivered to the liver throughout the process.

Serum estrogen levels can be utilized as a representation of measurement for hepatic stimulation only when the two techniques being compared use the same delivery mechanism and both have the same liver first-pass impact (e.g., two oral contraceptives). Thus, the representation of measurement will be faulty when comparing two totally different delivery systems, i.e., an oral to a transdermal method. Transdermal estrogen levels may not have a stronger hepatic impact than tablet levels. Transdermal estrogen probably does not boost liver estrogen absorption.

The hepatic exposure to estrogen that is caused by contraceptive pills is significantly more than what is indicated by blood estrogen levels. On the other hand, all of the estrogens to which the liver may be exposed are reflected in the serum levels while using transdermal devices.[15]

CURRENT STATUS OF CONTRACEPTIVE PATCHES

The new patches under clinical trials are grounded on changes, firstly, on lower estrogen exposure based on AUC and secondly with different progestins.

The first patch is a compact EE/gestodene (GSD) patch that is transparent and is now being researched in Europe. This patch is similar to the EE/norelgestromin patch, made from an adhesive polymer matrix diffusion-controlled drug delivery system; but, it has a two times smaller patch size. Here, norelgestromin is substituted with a more potent progestin called GSD, which has a higher skin penetration rate.[16]

Similarly, the second new patch is the EE/levonorgestrel (LNG) patch studies in the United States.

The third transdermal patch contains a delivery method that is regulated by the segmentation of a micro-reservoir. It provides a distribution of estradiol with dual-control mechanisms and levonorgestrel at constant rates (zero-order kinetics).[17]

FUTURE OF CONTRACEPTIVE PATCHES

Transdermal contraceptive patches have already established their ability to help women adhere more consistently to their use. As newer patches are developed with safer and lower doses of estrogen with or without different progestin, the essential demand of the once-a-week administration will lure new urgency in requirement to this delivery system.

Women worldwide find daily pill intake a burden and on the other hand find vaginal drug administration, intrauterine devices, or implants uncomfortable. These are the women for whom transdermal patches are an excellent choice, providing the hormonal contraceptives they desire which are safer and hassle-free.

KEY POINTS

- When it comes to combination hormonal birth control, transdermal contraceptive patches are more convenient to use than daily oral contraceptives.
- Numerous studies have indicated that women who use contraceptive patches are more likely to adhere to their chosen method than those who take pills.
- The most recent contraceptive patch was found to have side effects that were comparable to those seen with oral contraceptives.
- Patch application prevents hormone highs and lows caused by daily pill administration. This is one of many patch benefits.
- The elevated serum estrogen that occurs as a consequence of using the patch does

not, however, correlate to proportionally higher risks for venous thromboembolism.

- Newer versions of the patch, either progestin-only patches or patches with lower levels of EE estrogen, both have great potential as a better alternative contraceptive method in the future.

REFERENCES

1. Cerel-Suhl SL, Yeager BF. Update on oral contraceptive pills. Am Fam Phys.1999; 60(7): 2073-84.
2. NHS. (2021). Contraceptive patch: Your contraception guide. [online] Available from http://www.nhs.uk/Conditions/contraception-guide/Pages/contraceptive-patch.aspx [Last accessed November, 2022].
3. Potts RO, Lobo RA. Transdermal drug delivery: clinical considerations for the obstetrician-gynecologist. Obstet Gynecol. 2005;105(5 pt 1):953-61.
4. Graziottin A. A review of transdermal hormonal contraception: focus on the ethinylestradiol/norelgestromin contraceptive patch. Treat Endocrinol. 2006;5(6): 359-65.
5. Archer DF, Cullins V, Creasy GW, Fisher AC. The impact of improved compliance with a weekly contraceptive transdermal system (Ortho Evra) on contraceptive efficacy. Contraception. 2004;69(3):189-95.
6. Gallo MF, Grimes DA, Schulz KF. Skin patch and vaginal ring versus combined oral contraceptives for contraception. Cochrane Database Syst Rev. 2003;(1):CD003552.
7. Rubinstein ML, Halpern-Felsher BL, Irwin CE Jr. An evaluation of the use of the transdermal contraceptive patch in adolescents. J Adolesc Health. 2004;34(5):395-401.
8. Logsdon S, Richards J, Omar HA. Long-term evaluation of the use of the transdermal contraceptive patch in adolescents. Scientific World J. 2004;4:512-6.
9. Harel Z, Riggs S, Vaz R, Flanagan P, Dunn K, Harel D. Adolescents' experience with the combined estrogen and progestin transdermal contraceptive method Ortho Evra. J Pediatr Adolesc Gynecol. 2005;18(2): 85-90.
10. Archer DF, Bigrigg A, Smallwood GH, Shangold GA, Creasy GW, Fisher AC. Assessment of compliance with a weekly contraceptive patch (Ortho Evra™/Evra™) among North American women. Fertility and Sterility. 2002;77:27-31.
11. Bodner K, Bodner-Adler B, Grünberger W. Evaluation of the contraceptive efficacy, compliance, and satisfaction with the transdermal contraceptive patch system Evra: a comparison between adolescent and adult users. Arch Gynecol Obstet. 2011;283(3):525-30.
12. Zieman M, Guillebaud J, Weisberg E, Shangold GA, Fisher AC, Creasy GW. Contraceptive efficacy and cycle control with the Ortho Evra/Evra transdermal system: the analysis of pooled data. Fertil Steril. 2002;77(2 Suppl 2):S13-8.
13. Trussell J. Contraceptive failure in the United States. Contraception. 2011;83(5):397-404.
14. Zacur HA, Hedon B, Mansour D, Shangold GA, Fisher AC, Creasy GW. Integrated summary of Ortho Evra/Evra contraceptive patch adhesion in varied climates and conditions. Fertil Steril. 2002;77(2 suppl 2):S32-5.
15. Johnson JV, Lowell J, Badger G, Cushman M. The effects of oral and transdermal hormonal contraception on coagulation factors: a prospective, randomized, cross-over trial. Presented at: Society for Gynecologic Investigation. Toronto, ON, Canada, 22–25 March 2006.
16. Waellnitz K, Duijkers I, Klipping C, Rautenberg T, Rohde B, Zurth C. A two-centre, open label, randomised study of ovulation inhibition with three transdermal contraceptive patches, each containing different amounts of ethinyl estradiol and gestodene in healthy, young women. J Obstet Gynaecol. 2016;36(1):106-13.
17. Kaunitz AM, Portman D, Westhoff CL, Archer DF, Mishell DR Jr, Rubin A, et al. Low-dose levonorgestrel and ethinyl estradiol patch and pill: a randomized control trial. Obstet Gynecol. 2014;123(2 pt 1):295-303.

CHAPTER 7

Injectable Longer Action Reversible Contraception

Hafizur Rahman, Sivaranjani P

INTRODUCTION

Oral hormonal contraceptives are an effective short-acting contraception. Activity of these hormones could be prolonged by adding on an additional chemical group to form an ester. Injectable form of these compounds is slowly released into the systemic circulation, and thereby provides long-lasting activity. In 1950s, quite a number of esters of different estrogens and progestogens were synthesized and made up as microcrystalline suspensions. These injections are a method of longer action reversible contraception (LARC).

Injectable contraception is a highly effective form of contraception that has become acceptable all around the globe. More than 40 million women use injectable contraceptive to prevent conception.[1] Between 1995 and 2005, the use of injectable contraceptives doubled worldwide.[2] In sub-Saharan Africa more than one-third of the contraceptive users rely on injectable contraceptives.[3] Available injectable contraceptives are effective for 1–3 months and it leads to increase in the frequency of hospital visits.[4] The disadvantage of increased frequency of hospital visit leads to increased discontinuation rate despite its widespread use.[5] Injectable contraceptives with longer interval between the injections has better adherence and continuation rates than the one with shorter interval between the injections. The 1-year continuation rate for 3-monthly injectable contraceptive is better than a monthly injectable contraceptive.[6] This issue is combated by 6-monthly injectable contraceptives.

TYPES OF INJECTABLE CONTRACEPTIVES

Injectable contraceptives are mainly of two types:

1. Combined injectable contraceptives containing estrogen and progesterone-monthly injection.
2. Progesterone only injectable containing only synthetic progesterone.
   - Depot medroxyprogesterone acetate (DMPA)—every 3 monthly
   - Norethisterone enanthate—every 2 monthly
   - Levonorgestrel butanoate.

COMBINED INJECTABLE CONTRACEPTIVES

Combined injectable contraceptives (CICs) contain both estrogen and progesterone. These are developed to overcome the side effects of progesterone only formulations. The contraceptive effectiveness of CICs and progesterone only formulations is similar. It is administered every 28 days cycle.

Available formulations:
- Dihydroxyprogesterone acetophenide (also known as algestone acetophenide or alfasona) 75 mg and estradiol enanthate 5 mg.
- Dihydroxyprogesterone acetophenide 120 mg and estradiol enanthate 10 mg.
- Dihydroxyprogesterone acetophenide 150 mg and estradiol enanthate 10 mg.
- Dihydroxyprogesterone acetophenide 150 mg and estradiol benzoate 10 mg.
- Medroxyprogesterone acetate 25 mg and estradiol cypionate 5 mg—cyclofem.
- Norethisterone enanthate 50 mg and estradiol valerate 5 mg—mesigyna.
- Progesterone 50 mg and estradiol benzoate 5 mg.

Cyclofem and mesigyna are available in Asian and Latin American countries.[7] Cyclofem was introduced in the United States in the name of Lunelle but now it is no longer available.

Advantages

- With the added estrogen the menstrual cycles are more regular compare to progesterone only formulations.[8]
- Progesterone only formulations produce thin endometrium leading to irregular bleeding whereas estrogen component of CICs may build up the endometrium and thus regulate the bleeding patterns, mimicking the typical menstrual cycle.[9]
- There is more rapid return to fertility in CICs compare to progesterone only formulations.[9]

Disadvantages

- As it is a monthly injection, there is increased frequency of hospital visits.[9]
- The discontinuation rate is higher and the reasons being other than the bleeding disruptions.

PROGESTERONE ONLY INJECTABLE CONTRACEPTIVES

- Depot medroxyprogesterone acetate (DMPA)
- Norethisterone enanthate (NETEN)
- Levonorgestrel butanoate.

The duration of action is prolonged with the addition of either micronized aqueous solution or esterification.

Depot Medroxyprogesterone Acetate

Composition

Depot medroxyprogesterone acetate is an aqueous solution of microcrystal for depot injection of pregnane 17-α-hydroxyprogesterone-derivative progestin medroxyprogesterone acetate.

Mechanism of Action

Depot medroxyprogesterone acetate acts in the following way:
- Suppresses midcycle LH and FSH peak, thereby it prevents ovulation.
- Hypoestrogenic effect thickens the cervical mucus thereby prevents sperm ascend into the upper reproductive tract.
- Owing to the high progesterone and low estrogen, endometrium thins and becomes unfavorable for implantation.

Contraceptive Benefits

- *Effectiveness:* Highly effective, reversible, long-acting, progesterone only contraceptive.[10] Provides immediate contraception with failure rate lower than that of oral contraceptives with typical use.[10] The use failure rate is 0.3% which is lower than 0.5% in female sterilization, 0.8% in IUCD. (WHO Family Planning: A Global Handbook for Providers).

- User friendly, avoids inconvenience of daily use and anxiety of backup method.
- Completely reversible
- Does not interfere with sexual intercourse.
- Does not require pelvic examination prior to administration.
- Efficacy not compromised with BMI
- Can be used in situation where estrogen is contraindicated like in women >35 years who smoke and in obesity.
- *DMPA and medical abortion:* Providing DMPA at the time of aspiration abortion increases the use of DMPA.[11] There are concerns about using progesterone only contraception while administration mifepristone for medical abortion as DMPA could counteract the abortifacient effect of mifepristone. 96% of the women who received DMPA on the day of mifepristone administration completed abortion compared to 100% who received etonogestrel implant.[12]
- Depot medroxyprogesterone acetate used in postpartum moms between 6 weeks and 6 months even if the mother is exclusively breastfeeding and menstrual cycles not returned.
- Can be used by women of all age and parity.

Noncontraceptive Benefits

- Thirty-nine percent reduction in the risk of epithelial ovarian cancer.[13]
- Decreases dysmenorrhea and premenstrual symptoms.
- Protective against endometrial cancer
- Alleviates the symptoms of endometriosis.
- Improves anemia by reducing the menstrual blood loss and by causing amenorrhea.
- Reduce incidence of benign breast disease and ovarian cyst.
- Overall incidence of pelvic inflammatory disease (PID) is reduced.
- Reduces the risk of sickle-cell crisis in women with sickle-cell anemia.
- As it supresses ovulation, it protects against ectopic pregnancy.
- Helps to prevent uterine tumors (fibroids).

Disadvantages

- Any side effects to be tolerated once DMPA is administered till the progesterone effect weans off.
- Menstrual irregularities and amenorrhea.
- 40–50% increased risk of HIV compared to non-contraceptive users.[14] And the mechanism are modification in the protective epithelial barrier of the female genital tract, modification of the vaginal microflora, alteration in the genital immunity and change in HIV-1 target cell activation.[15] Hypoestrogenic effect of DMPA causes vaginal thinning.[16] Increased risk of HIV acquisition in DMPA users compared to NEAN users.[17] In 2017 WHO changed MEC DMPA in the group of people with increased risk of HIV acquisition from category 1 to category 2.
- Its use has been associated with decrease in the bone mineral density.[18] Estrogen downregulates the osteoclastic activity thereby controlling the bone resorption.[19] Medroxyprogesterone acetate inhibits gonadotropin secretion thus decreases the ovarian estradiol production.[20] WHO, ACOG, and RCOG none recommend initiation or duration of use considering the skeletal hazards or recommend routine BMD in DMPA users.[21] But, the Food and Drug Administration (FDA) indicated that DMPA can be used for >2 years only if other contraceptive methods are contraindicated.[22]
- DMPA suppresses both natural and acquired immunity because of its greater affinity with glucocorticoid receptor which signals T-cell apoptosis.[23]

- Side effects of DMPA is due to its androgenic and/or glucocorticoid activities and are dose dependant. Lowering the dose could improve the safety profile of DMPA. Subcutaneous dose of DMPA has greater efficacy than IM DMPA with 30% lower dose.[24]
- Weight gain, bloating, depression, and mastalgia.
- Decreased libido and dry vagina.

Depot Medroxyprogesterone Acetate Subcutaneous

The rate of absorption is slower in subcutaneous than the intramuscular formulation.[25] The contraceptive efficacy and tolerability profile are similar or even better with depot medroxyprogesterone acetate subcutaneous (DMPA-SC).[26] DMPA-SC was introduced earliest in four countries, Burkina Faso, Senegal, Uganda, and Niger.[27] DMPA-SC (104 mg) is of same efficacy as that of DMPA-IM but with 30% lower dose.[27] Injection site reaction is more with DMPA-SC than DMPA-IM.[24] The depression and mood changes was similar in both the DMPA-IM and DMPA-SC group.[28] Irregular cycle decreased over the period of usage whereas the incidence of amenorrhea increased.[29] The discontinuation rate with DMPA-IM is 40–50% at the end of 12 months whereas it has found that there is 50% increase in the continuation rate in DMPA-SC self-injectors compared to provider administered injections.[30]

Contraindications

Absolute contraindications:

- Diagnosed pregnancy
- Undiagnosed abnormal vaginal bleeding
- Diagnosed or suspected breast cancer
- Active liver disease or jaundice
- Active thrombophlebitis
- Sensitivity to DMPA.

Relative contraindications:

- Severe depression
- Migraine
- Abnormal glucose tolerance test
- Hyperlipidemia (LDL >160)

When to start DMPA?

If the woman is reasonably sure that she is not pregnant, DMPA injection can be started any time. **Table 1** lists different phases of women, when one can start the first dose of DMPA injection to be an effective contraceptive method.[19]

Norethisterone Enanthate

It is an ester and prodrug of norethisterone.[31] The effect of intramuscular injection of 50–200 mg lasts for 11–52 days.[32] NETE has strong progesterogenic activity with weak androgenic and estrogenic activity.[33] The weak estrogenic activity is due to its metabolite, ethinyl estradiol. The side effects are mastalgia, headache, depression, irregular menstruation, and injection site pain.[34] It can cause birth defects if used during pregnancy.[31]

Levonorgestrel Butanoate

Levonorgestrel butanoate is esterified analog of levonorgestrel. This butanoate ester prolongs the half-life. The formulation is aqueous suspension that can be injected intramuscularly. The available doses are 5 mg, 10 mg, and 50 mg. 5 mg and 10 mg have the duration of action for 3 months[35] whereas 50 mg has 6 months duration of action.[36] Because of its lower dosage, the progesteronic side effects like hypogonadism and amenorrhea are lesser compared to DMPA and the return of fertility is rapid.[37]

TABLE 1: Different phases of women.

Situation	*Timing to start*
When women having menstrual cycles or want to switch from a nonhormonal method	Can be started any day within 7 days—no additional precaution needed
While switching from a hormonal method	Can be started immediately, if it is reasonably certain that the woman is not pregnant. No need for a backup method
Postpartum within 6 months, breastfeeding	• Wait first 6 weeks postpartum and then start DMPA • Between 6 weeks and 6 months can be started anytime if she is exclusively breastfeeding—no need for a backup method. However, if partially breastfeeding, can be started at any time, it is reasonably certain that the woman is not pregnant
Postpartum—beyond 6 months	Can be started at any time, if her menstruation has not resumed and if it is sure that the woman is not pregnant. Use backup method for the first 7 days after DMPA injection
Postpartum not breastfeeding	Within 4 weeks after giving birth can be started at any time. No need for a backup method. After 4 weeks can be started any time, if her monthly bleeding has not returned and the woman is certain of not pregnant-need backup for 7 days
After miscarriage or abortion	Can be started immediately after abortion or within 7 days of first- or second-trimester miscarriage/abortion, with no need for a backup method. After >7 days of first- or second-trimester miscarriage/abortion, can be started anytime if it is reasonably certain that woman is not pregnant-backup needed for first 7 days of injection
After taking emergency contraceptive pills (ECPs)	DMPA can be started on the same day when ECP taken. If started within 7 days of period, an additional backup method for first 7 days is recommended

(DMPA: depot medroxyprogesterone acetate)

KEY POINTS

- Injectable contraception is a highly effective and popular form of contraception all around the globe.
- Combined injectable and progesterone only injectable are the two types of injectable contraceptives.
- Combined injectable contraceptives contains both estrogen and progesterone and it is monthly injections.
- Depot medroxyprogesterone acetate, norethisterone enanthate, and levonorgestrel butanoate are progesterone only injectables.
- The use failure rate of DMPA is 0.3%.
- DMPA is protective against epithelial ovarian carcinoma and endometrial carcinoma.
- DMPA can be given in postabortal state and postpartum.
- DMPA is associated with increased risk of HIV and reduce bone mineral density.
- DMPA-SC has similar efficacy as that of DMPA-IM with 30% lower dosage.
- The effect of intramuscular injection of NETE, 50–200 mg lasts for 11–52 days.
- The available doses of levonorgestrel butanoate are 5 mg, 10 mg, and 50 mg. The effect for 5 mg and 10 mg is 3 months whereas it is 6 months for 50 mg.

REFERENCES

1. United Nations Population Division |Department of Economic and Social Affairs [Internet]. [cited 2022 Jul 27]. [online] Available from: https://www.un.org/en/development/desa/population/publications/family/contraceptive-wallchart-2011.asp [Last accessed November, 2022].
2. Expanding services for injectables. [Internet]. [cited 2022 Jul 27]. [online] Available from: https://www.cabdirect.org/cabdirect/abstract/20073221843 [Last accessed November, 2022].
3. Injectable contraception provided by community-based health workers: one important step toward meeting unmet need. Glob Heal Sci Pract [Internet]. 2013;1(3):287.
4. Lakha F, Henderson C, Glasier A. The acceptability of self-administration of subcutaneous Depo-Provera. Contraception [Internet]. 2005;72(1):14-8.
5. Baumgartner JN, Morroni C, Mlobeli RD, Otterness C, Myer L, Janowitz B, et al. Timeliness of contraceptive reinjections in South Africa and its relation to unintentional discontinuation. Int Fam Plan Perspect [Internet]. 2007 Jun [cited 2022 Jul 27];33(2): 66-74.
6. González-Arenas A, Hansberg-Pastor V, Hernández-Hernández OT, González-García TK, Henderson-Villalpando J, Lemus-Hernández D, et al. Estradiol increases cell growth in human astrocytoma cell lines through ERα activation and its interaction with SRC-1 and SRC-3 coactivators. Biochim Biophys Acta [Internet]. 2012;1823(2):379-86.
7. D'Arcangues C. Comparative study of the effects of two once-a-month injectable contraceptives (Cyclofem® and Mesigyna®) and one oral contraceptive (Ortho-Novum 1/35®) on coagulation and fibrinolysis. Contraception. 2003;68(3):159-76.
8. Gallo MF, Grimes DA, Lopez LM, Schulz KF, D'Arcangues C. Combination injectable contraceptives for contraception. Cochrane Database Syst Rev [Internet]. 2008;2008(4).
9. Kaunitz AM. Injectable contraception. New and existing options. Obstet Gynecol Clin North Am [Internet]. 2000;27(4):741-80.
10. Allen RH, Cwiak CA, Kaunitz AM. Contraception in women over 40 years of age. CMAJ [Internet]. 2013;185(7):565-73.
11. Hathaway M, Torres L, Vollett-Krech J, Wohltjen H. Increasing LARC utilization: any woman, any place, any time. Clin Obstet Gynecol [Internet]. 2014;57(4):718-30.
12. Park J, Robinson N, Wessels U, Turner J, Geller S. Progestin-based contraceptive on the same day as medical abortion. Int J Gynaecol Obstet [Internet]. 2016;133(2):217.
13. Wilailak S, Vipupinyo C, Suraseranivong V, Chotivanich K, Kietpeerakool C, Tanapat Y, et al. Depot medroxyprogesterone acetate and epithelial ovarian cancer: a multicentre case-control study. BJOG [Internet]. 2012;119(6):672-7.
14. Morrison CS, Chen PL, Kwok C, Baeten JM, Brown J, Crook AM, et al. Hormonal Contraception and the Risk of HIV Acquisition: An Individual Participant Data Meta-analysis. PLOS Med [Internet]. 2015;12(1):e1001778.
15. Wessels JM, Lajoie J, Hay Cooper MIJ, Omollo K, Felker AM, Vitali D, et al. Medroxyprogesterone acetate alters the vaginal microbiota and microenvironment in women and increases susceptibility to HIV-1 in humanized mice. Dis Model Mech [Internet]. 2019;12(10).
16. Morrison CS, Turner AN, Jones LSB. Highly effective contraception and acquisition of HIV and other sexually transmitted infections. Best Pract Res Clin Obstet Gynaecol [Internet]. 2009;23(2):263-84.
17. Polis CB, Curtis KM, Hannaford PC, Phillips SJ, Chipato T, Kiarie JN, et al. An updated systematic review of epidemiological evidence on hormonal contraceptive methods and HIV acquisition in women. AIDS [Internet]. 2016;30(17):2665-83.
18. Curtis KM, Martins SL. Progestogen-only contraception and bone mineral density: a systematic review. Contraception [Internet]. 2006;73(5):470-87.
19. Family Planning Masterclass: Evidence-based Answers to 1000 Questions - Google Books [Internet]. [cited 2022 Jul 28]. [online] Available from: https://books.google.co.in/books?id=8Hv4gdmqPCAC&pg=PA518&lpg=PA518&dq=%5D+Gbolade+BA.+Depo-Provera+and+bone+density.+J+Fa

m+Plann+Reprod+Health+Care+2002;28:7-11&source=bl&ots=8AaibFlzmV&sig=ACfU3U3e3ZkbWncyXh_d6StBeVcqTe56fw&hl=en&sa=X&ved= 2ahUKEwi5gv3rspj5AhWxpVYBHT4MDKwQ6AF6BAgDEAM#v=onepage&q=%5D Gbolade BA. Depo-Provera and bone density. J Fam Plann Reprod Health Care 2002%3B28%3A7-11&f=false [Last accessed November, 2022].
20. Clark MK, Sowers MF, Levy BT, Tenhundfeld P. Magnitude and variability of sequential estradiol and progesterone concentrations in women using depot medroxyprogesterone acetate for contraception. Fertil Steril [Internet]. 2001;75(5):871-7.
21. ACOG practice bulletin. No. 73: Use of hormonal contraception in women with coexisting medical conditions. Obstet Gynecol [Internet]. 2006;107(6):1453-72.
22. Paschall S, Kaunitz AM. Depo-Provera and skeletal health: a survey of Florida obstetrics and gynecologist physicians. Contraception [Internet]. 2008;78(5):370-6.
23. Hapgood JP, Ray RM, Govender Y, Avenant C, Tomasicchio M. Differential Glucocorticoid Receptor-Mediated Effects on Immunomodulatory Gene Expression by Progestin Contraceptives: Implications for HIV-1 Pathogenesis. Am J Reprod Immunol. 2014;71(6):505-12.
24. Kaunitz AM, Darney PD, Ross D, Wolter KD, Speroff L. Subcutaneous DMPA vs. intramuscular DMPA: a 2-year randomized study of contraceptive efficacy and bone mineral density. Contraception [Internet]. 2009; 80(1):7-17.
25. Jain J, Dutton C, Nicosia A, Wajszczuk C, Bode FR, Mishell DR. Pharmacokinetics, ovulation suppression and return to ovulation following a lower dose subcutaneous formulation of Depo-Provera. Contraception [Internet]. 2004;70(1):11-8.
26. Jain J, Jakimiuk AJ, Bode FR, Ross D, Kaunitz AM. Contraceptive efficacy and safety of DMPA-SC. Contraception [Internet]. 2004; 70(4):269-75.
27. Cole K, Saad A. The coming-of-age of subcutaneous injectable contraception. Glob Heal Sci Pract. 2018;6(1):1-5.
28. Weissman MM, Bland RC, Canino GJ, Faravelli C, Greenwald S, Hwu HG, et al. The cross-national epidemiology of panic disorder. Arch Gen Psychiatry. 1997;54(4):305-9.
29. Belsey EM, Task Force on Long-Acting Systemic Agents for Fertility Regulation. Vaginal bleeding patterns among women using one natural and eight hormonal methods of contraception. Contraception [Internet]. 1988;38(2):181-206.
30. Burke HM, Chen M, Buluzi M, Fuchs R, Wevill S, Venkatasubramanian L, et al. Effect of self-administration versus provider-administered injection of subcutaneous depot medroxyprogesterone acetate on continuation rates in Malawi: a randomised controlled trial. Lancet Glob Heal [Internet]. 2018;6(5):e568-78.
31. Wu L, Janagam DR, Mandrell TD, Johnson JR, Lowe TL. Long-acting injectable hormonal dosage forms for contraception. Pharm Res [Internet]. 2015;32(7):2180-91.
32. Davis ME, Wied GL. 17-alpha-HYDROXY-PROGESTERONE acetate; an effective progestational substance on oral administration. J Clin Endocrinol Metab. 1957;17(10):1237-44.
33. Shapiro S. Oral oestrogen-progestagen contraceptives, menopausal treatment, and cancer. Lancet Oncol [Internet]. 2005;6(10): 736; author reply 737.
34. Melis GB, Strigini F, Fruzzetti F, Paoletti AM, Rainer E, Düsterberg B, et al. Norethisterone enanthate as an injectable contraceptive in puerperal and non-puerperal women. Contraception. 1981;23(1):77-88.
35. Toppozada M. The clinical use of monthly injectable contraceptive preparations. Obs Gynecol Surv. 1977;32(6):335-47.
36. Details for: Varney's midwifery: WHO Searo Library catalog [Internet]. [cited 2022 Jul 28]. [online] Available from: https://libraryopac.searo.who.int/cgi-bin/koha/opac-detail.pl?biblionumber=7856 [Last accessed November, 2022].
37. Senanayake PP. Atlas of Contraception. [Internet]. CRC Press; 2019 [cited 2022 Jul 28]. [online] Available from: https://www.routledge.com/Atlas-of-Contraception/Senanayake-Potts/p/book/9780367387488 [Last accessed November, 2022].

CHAPTER 8

Intrauterine Contraceptive Devices

Indranil Dutta

INTRODUCTION

Intrauterine devices (IUDs) are one of the most widely used form of contraception currently available in market in private as well as government channels. Other forms of sterilization have comparable failure rates to IUDs.

Commonly used IUDs are copper-containing IUD, and levonorgestrel-containing IUDs. Copper-containing IUDs are widely available throughout the country in Government Channels particularly as the part of postpartum intrauterine contraceptive device (PPIUCD) project in which they are provided free to patients immediately post deliveries.

These IUDs are also known as long-acting reversible contraception (LARC) and have good acceptability rates.

PAST

History leads us to the first of IUDs which was developed way back in 1909. A renowned German Physician Richard Ricter of Walenberg had discovered device which was made of silk-worm gut.[1] This material was the main core and was encircled by alloy of copper, nickel, and zinc, and it was working well at those times to prevent pregnancies. The role of elastic metallic rings as IUDs was brought forward by Tenrey Ota in 1934.[2]

Intrauterine devices in 1950s were popularized by Jack Lippes in the United States. His Lippe's loop became one of the most popular *first generation IUDs.* "T"-shaped design was popularly as modern methods of IUD by 1960s. However, the US physician Howard Tatum was the one who found out the advantage of T shape which would be beneficial to reduce expulsion.

Tatum and Jaime Zipper had discovered the advantages of effective spermicidal and had developed first Copper IUD, TCu200 (*second-generation IUDs*), and further modifications by Tatum was mainly responsible for TCu380a which nowadays is one of the most widely preferred copper IUDs.

The creation of hormonal IUDs (*third-generation IUDs*) was invented around 1960s to 1970s. The rampant problems which were associated with Copper IUDs that increased bleeding and this problem was addressed well with development of hormonal IUDs. The commercially available hormonal IUDs named as "Mirena" is still being used widely all over the world.

In past, uterine width has been attributed to be the main criteria for shaping the IUDs, but various studies around the world have shown that width may vary in people especially it may be more narrow in nulliparous women.

INDICATIONS FOR INSERTION

Two primary types of IUDs have different indications of use particularly also to note that both can be used for contraception purpose.

Levonorgestrel-containing IUDs are available in different strengths around the world but popularly in strength of 52 mg. Apart from the use of contraception, it can also be used for treatment of menorrhagia. Use is limited to time of 5 years.[2]

One of the main advantages of copper IUD TCu380a was that it was approved for use up to 10 years. It also had a huge advantage of being used as an emergency contraception up to 5 days post unprotected intercourse.

Levonorgestrel-releasing intrauterine device (LNG-IUD) also has advantage of being used as postpartum IUD and could be placed within cavity 10 minutes of delivery of the placenta, delayed postpartum within 4–6 weeks of delivery and postabortion.[3]

Postabortion insertion also can be done following abortion or miscarriage.

INDICATION FOR REMOVAL

- Patient wants pregnancy
- Abnormal menstrual bleeding
- Discomfort
- Excessive vaginal bleeding
- Pain.[4]

CONTRAINDICATIONS

Common Contraindications for Intrauterine Devices

- Pregnancy
- Sexually transmitted diseases (STDs) at the time of insertion
- Confirmed malignancy
- Acute pelvic inflammatory disease (PID)
- Abnormal uterine bleeding (AUB)
- Device causing hypersensitivity
- Congenital uterine abnormality.

Additional Contraindications: Levonorgestrel-releasing Intrauterine System

- Active liver disease
- Breast malignancy or progestin sensitive cancer
- Liver malignancy or tumors.

Additional Contraindications: Copper T

- Wilson's disease
- Sensitivity to copper.

PROCEDURE

Setup and Instruments Required for Inserting Intrauterine Device

- OPD sterile setup
- Cusco's speculum
- Gloves
- Antiseptic solutions
- Uterine sound
- Uterine dilators
- Scissors
- Anesthesia support system (in case deciding to perform under paracervical block).

Who can conduct?

Any trained healthcare provider.

PREPARATION

Firstly, choice of patient is most important keeping in mind the contraindications in particular. Patient counseling is most important before the procedure is being conducted.

The safety and acceptability of LARC should be broadly discussed with patients. Government of India supplies IUD free of cost at most of the healthcare facilities. If there is no such contraindication then IUDs can be preferred choice.[5-7]

Consent of the patient and her husband is most important step. Postconsent ruling out active pregnancy is important followed by assessment of patient.[8]

Sexual intercourse history is very important as sometimes patient may have irregular cycles and may give vague history as such. If criteria are not met then additional safety can be given in form of other contraceptives till the time she is fit for the IUD insertion or falls in criteria.

Sexually transmitted disorders have to be ruled out prior to insertion.[9] Patients who have not been screened should be screened prior but that should not be the hindrance for insertion.

A number of discussions have been done around the world regarding use of pain killer medicines prior to the procedure but same does not have a additional benefit.[10] It was detrimental because of delaying insertion of IUD, but tablets like misoprostol helped in insertions sometimes particularly in those patients with previous history of difficult insertion.

TECHNIQUE

- Take proper consent from patient and her husband.
- Take proper history of any active infection.
- Rule out pregnancy.
- Positioning to dorsal lithotomy.
- Bimanual examination to check ante- or retroversion of uterus.
- Insert speculum and clean cervix preferably with betadine.
- Hold cervix with tenaculum and determine length of uterine cavity using uterine sound.
- Dilators may be used if at all required.
- Check IUD package for expiry or any other defects.
- Insert IUD in the cavity in an aseptic manner.
- Counsel patient regarding checking the string at few intervals.
- Call patient for follow up after 6 weeks.

COMPLICATIONS

- Expulsion
- Displacement of IUD
- Uterine perforation
- Bleeding
- Vasovagal symptoms with bradycardia
- Pelvic inflammatory disease
- Small probability of pregnancy.

FUTURE

Newer IUDs are currently under development, they have been modified to suit patient and physician satisfaction.[11] Some are under development or have been introduced already.

Cu Safe 300

It was mainly designed to reduce side effects such as expulsion, associated bleeding, and sometimes pain. Another important change is the frame of device is smaller. Side arms are thinner which allows easy insertion. Recommended life span is 5 years.

Fincoid-350

This device has a plastic skeleton comprising two parts: curved horizontal arms and a copper-coated vertical stem. The horizontal arms lock into groove on the vertical stem. Thus, enabling the easy movement of joint and also has advantage of being able to constrict and expand with uterine contractions. Mainly this device also resists expulsion.

Gynefix

Frameless intrauterine system (IUS) was developed to reduce failures related to traditional IUDs, i.e., pain, bleeding, and expulsions. It consists of six 5-mm copper sleeves with an effective copper surface area of 330 mm^2, fixed on the length of semi-rigid suture thread. Most important point here is that the knot is to be implanted into the myometrium of uterine fundus.[12]

INTRACERVICAL FIXING DEVICE

The device is composed of rod-shaped, copper-coated polyethylene frame that is 4 cm long, with a 5-mm projection at the distal end. This projection enables the device to be anchored to inner cervical wall using a modified tenaculum.

Advantage of the system is the insertion procedure is not blind; device is less likely to have spotting, bleeding, and pain.[13]

SUMMARY

To summarize IUDs, there have been the mainstay in reducing unwanted pregnancies. But the main success lies within the fact that the device is reliable, it is very cheap and sometimes even free in government channels and also very effective in its wide use among population.

But, some amount of negativity has surrounded IUD use due to unexpected bleeding issues. Newer IUDs are being developed and studied around the world for better patient and doctor compliance. And also to mention the fact that CuT380A remains one the widely used IUD around the world and more studies are required to corroborate the same.

REFERENCES

1. Thiery M. Pioneers of the intrauterine device. Eur J Contracep Reprod Health Care. 2006;2(1):15-3.
2. Apter D, Gemzell-Danielsson K, Hauck B, Rosen K, Zurth C. Pharmacokinetics of two low-dose levonorgestrel-releasing intrauterine systems and effects on ovulation rate and cervical function: pooled analyses of phase II and III studies. Fertil Steril. 2014;101(6):1656-62.e1-4.
3. Chen BA, Reeves MF, Hayes JL, Hohmann HL, Perriera LK, Creinin MD. Postplacental or delayed insertion of the levonorgestrel intrauterine device after vaginal delivery: a randomized controlled trial. Obstet Gynecol. 2010;116(5):1079-87.
4. Strasser J, Borkowski L, Couillard M, Allina A, Wood SF. Access to removal of long-acting reversible contraceptive methods is an essential component of high-quality contraceptive care. Womens Health Issues. 2017; 27(3):253-5.
5. Boateng J, Chi IC, Jones DB. An evaluation of six new intrauterine devices. Adv Contracept. 1994;10:57-70.
6. Ota T. A study on the birth control with an intrauterine instrument. Jpn; J Obstet Gynecol. 1934;17:210-4.
7. Lanzola EL, Ketvertis K. Intrauterine Device. [Updated 2022 Jul 4]. In: StatPearls [Internet]. Treasure Island (FL): StatPearls Publishing; 2022. [online] Available from: https://www.ncbi.nlm.nih.gov/books/NBK557403 [Last accessed November, 2022].
8. Min J, Buckel C, Secura GM, Peipert JF, Madden T. Performance of a checklist to exclude pregnancy at the time of contraceptive initiation among women with a negative urine pregnancy test. Contraception. 2015;91(1):80-4.
9. Committee on Practice Bulletins-Gynecology, Long-Acting Reversible Contraception Work Group. Practice bulletin no. 186: Long-acting reversible contraception: implants and intrauterine devices. Obstet Gynecol. 2017; 130(5):e251-69.
10. Lopez LM, Bernholc A, Zeng Y, Allen RH, Bartz D, O'Brien PA, et al. Interventions for pain with intrauterine device insertion. Cochrane Database Syst Rev. 2015;(7): CD007373.
11. Suhonen S, Holmstrom T, Lahteenmaki P. Three-year follow-up of the use of a levonorgestrel releasing intrauterine system in hormone replacement therapy. Acta Obstet Gynecol Scand. 1997;76:145-50.
12. Rosenberg MJ, Foldesy R, Mishell DR Jr, Speroff L, Waugh MS, Burkman R. Performance of the TCu380A and Cu-Fix IUDs in an international randomized trial. Contraception. 1996;53:197-203.
13. International Study Group on Intrauterine Drug Delivery. The GyneFix® implant systems for interval, postabortal and postpartum contraception: a significant advance in long-term reversible contraception. Eur J Contracept Reprod Health Care. 1997;2:1-13.

CHAPTER 9

Spermicides

Sonali Deshpande, Apurva S Sholapure

INTRODUCTION

Spermicide is used to prevent pregnancy by destroying the sperm before sexual contact. Because of this, sperms are often unable to penetrate because they are unable to swim through the cervix as easily. The spermicidal substance is a chemical that eliminates sperm and other STD-causing microorganisms. Additionally, as a supplementary form of action, some delivery bases physically block the cervix to stop sperm and pathogens from entering the uterus. The membrane of the sperm or pathogen is the target of most spermicides, which are typically surfactants.

They are under the category of fourth-tier contraceptive techniques in terms of effectiveness **(Fig. 1)**.

HISTORY

The use of spermicide is first mentioned in the Kahun Papyrus, an Egyptian record from around 1850 BCE. It is characterized as a mixture of fermented dough and crocodile feces. It has been hypothesized that the dung's spermicidal properties stem from its acidic pH. Using quinine sulfate and cocoa butter, English pharmacist Walter Rendell developed the first spermicidal suppository in 1885. Nonoxynol-9, one of the most effective spermicidal chemicals developed in the 1950s, is still available in the United Kingdom via prescription.[1]

CHEMICAL NATURE AND TYPES

Spermicides consist of a spermicidal chemical and a delivery base. Nonoxynol-9 (N-9),

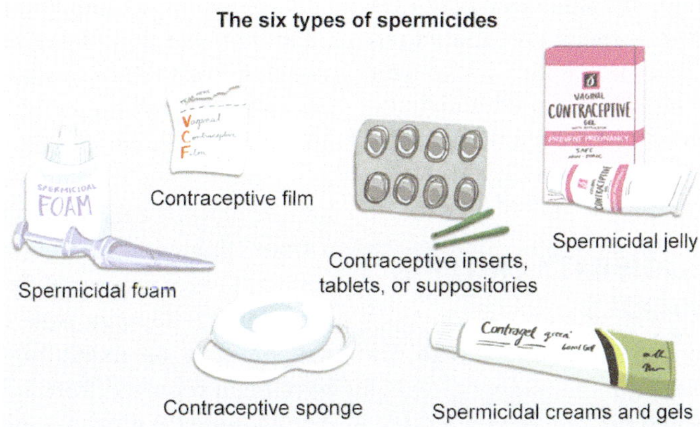

Fig. 1: Types of spermicides.

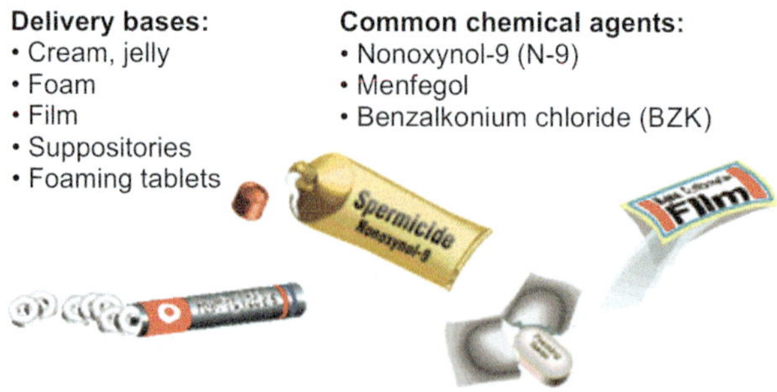

Fig. 2: Spermicides: Delivery bases and chemical agents.

menfegol, and benzalkonium chloride are the three spermicidal substances that are most commonly employed nowadays **(Fig. 2)**.

EFFECTIVENESS

"Typical use of failure rate: 21%"[2]

"Spermicides have a typical user failure rate of 21% and condoms 12%; combined, the 1st year probability of failure among typical users is 2.5%".[3]

The assumption of independence is likely high under ideal use when there is a proper use for every act of intercourse, and efficacy would be as high as steroidal implants.[3]

Effectiveness depends on the user.[4]

When spermicides do not seem to be used with every act of sex, the risk of pregnancy is highest. On average, the failure rate is 21 pregnancies out of every 100 women during the 1st year. This means that 79 out of every 100 women who use spermicides will not get pregnant. 16 pregnancies were discovered per 100 women who used spermicides over the course of the 1st year when administered correctly with every act of sexual activity. Once spermicide use has been discontinued, there is no delay in the recovery of fertility.

MEDICAL ELIGIBILITY CRITERIA FOR SPERMICIDES

Any woman may use spermicides, with the exception of those who:

- Are at an elevated risk of contracting HIV
- Be HIV positive.

CORRECT USE OF SPERMICIDES (FIGS. 3A TO G)

When injected high in the vagina, close to the cervix, spermicides provide the highest level of contraceptive protection. There is no downtime with topical treatments such as foams, jellies, and lotions because they go to work as soon as they are applied. There is a 5- to 15-minute waiting period associated with the use of suppositories, tablets, and films. After being implanted, spermicides have an effective time period of 1–2 hours. Creams, jellies, and foam all require an applicator for proper use. Load the applicator up with the jelly and the cream by squeezing the two together. Shaking foam containers is necessary for loading the applicator correctly. Manual insertion of the vaginal canal is required for suppositories, tablets, and film. Females using spermicidal products should wash their hands well before and after use, and should also use a sterile applicator. Given the variety of products on the market, it is important to have specific instructions for each application. The film should be folded in half and inserted using dry hands to prevent it from clinging to the fingers instead of the cervix. If there are many sexual interactions happening at the same time, more spermicide will need to be used. No adverse effects have been reported from using this product during menstruation. For best effectiveness, a spermicide should be used in conjunction

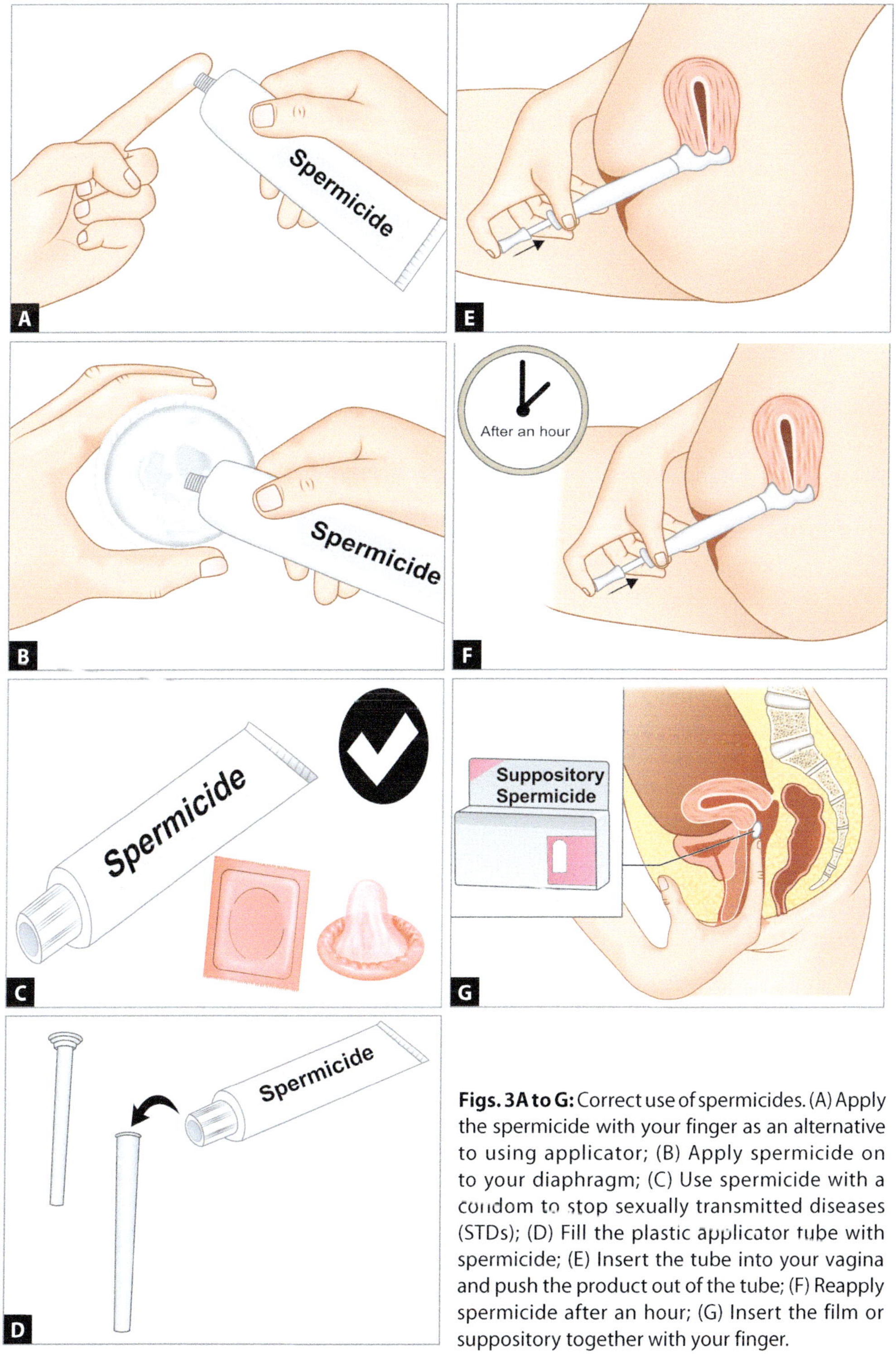

Figs. 3A to G: Correct use of spermicides. (A) Apply the spermicide with your finger as an alternative to using applicator; (B) Apply spermicide on to your diaphragm; (C) Use spermicide with a condom to stop sexually transmitted diseases (STDs); (D) Fill the plastic applicator tube with spermicide; (E) Insert the tube into your vagina and push the product out of the tube; (F) Reapply spermicide after an hour; (G) Insert the film or suppository together with your finger.

with another barrier method. After having sex, a lady should wait at least 6 hours before douching.

Advantages

- Total control over how it is used.
- Can be used on its own.
- There is no requirement of any prior assessment.
- Boosts lubrication.
- Does not include hormones.
- Rarely do side effects occur.
- Accessible without a prescription and reasonably priced.
- Can be inserted before the appointed time without preventing intercourse.

Disadvantages

- Planning is required, and availability is required during sexual activity.
- Repeat insertions at least once an hour.
- Does not offer STD protection.
- Not as efficient as other approaches.
- Infection of the urinary tract, itchiness, or allergies are possible side effects.
- Nonoxynol-9 consumption over time may raise the risk of contracting HIV.

CORRECTING MISUNDERSTANDINGS ABOUT SPERMICIDES[5]

- Do not protect against sexually transmitted infections (STIs).
- Do not make women bleed or reduce their vaginal secretions when having sex.
- Do not result in birth abnormalities or cervical cancer.
- Do not alter or lessen either men's or women's drive or pleasure.
- Do not stop the monthly bleeding in women.

FUTURE ASPECTS OF SPERMICIDE

A good preparation for its users, especially women who can use it as per their own preferences, would meet the following criteria. It should have a quick and irreversible effect on the sperm, not irritate the vaginal or penile mucosa, not harm the developing fetus, not have any adverse side effects, and not be absorbed into the body. Therefore, studies of currently under development spermicidal medicines should be evaluated in light of the above considerations.[6]

EVIDENCE

1. Grimes DA, Lopez LM, Raymond EG, Halpern V, Nanda K, Schulz KF. Spermicide used alone for contraception. Cochrane Database Syst Rev. 2013;9:CD005218.
2. Cook LA, Nanda K, Grimes DA, Lopez LM. Diaphragm versus diaphragm with spermicides for contraception. Cochrane Database Syst Rev. 2003;1:CD002031.

REFERENCES

1. "https://web.archive.org/web/20060926032018/http:/www.contraceptiononline.org/contrareport/article01.cfm?art=93"" Evolution and Revolution: The Past, Present, and Future of Contraception". Contraception Online (Baylor College of Medicine). 10 (6). February 2000. Archived from: "http://www.contraceptiononline.org/contrareport/article01.cfm?art=93"the original on September 26, 2006
2. https://www.cdc.gov/reproductivehealth/contraception/index.htm
3. Kestelman P, Trussell J. Efficacy of the simultaneous use of condoms and spermicides. Fam Plann Perspect. 1991;23(5):226-7, 232. PMID: 1743276.

4. https://fphandbook.org/chapter-16-spermicides-and-diaphragms
5. Family Planning: A Global Handbook for Providers (2022). Chapter 16: Correcting Misunderstandings—Spermicides Family Planning (fphandbook.org). [online] Available from: https://fphandbook.org/ correcting-misunderstandings-spermicides [Last accessed November, 2022].
6. Williams Gynecology, 3e Hoffman BL, Schorge JO, Bradshaw KD, Halvorson LM, Schaffer JI, Corton MM. Hoffman B.L., & Schorge J.O., & Bradshaw K.D., & Halvorson L.M., & Schaffer J.I., & Corton M.M.(Eds.),Eds. Barbara L.

CHAPTER 10

Female Barrier Contraceptive Methods

Sonali Deshpande, Apurva S Sholapure

INTRODUCTION

Uncontrolled human population growth is the greatest threat to our species' survival. Overpopulation is currently a major problem, and the only solution is to use contraception to reduce the human population.

Maybe population control is always necessary to ensure the sustainability of the ecosystem. Nature will take care of it for us in the worst conceivable way if we do not.

In order to curb population growth, there are now a variety of effective contraceptives to choose from.

Nowadays, techniques are sorted in accordance with how well they work **(Table 1)**.[1]

FEMALE BARRIER METHODS (FIG. 1)

Female condoms, cervical caps, vaginal diaphragms, and vault caps are a few of these.

Female Condom

Introduction

Male condoms are the most successful form of birth control, but female condoms are considered "third-tier" because of their low success rate (barrier methods). Thin and flexible synthetic latex, or latex is used to make condoms for women. This is achieved through the formation of a physical barrier that borders the vagina, seals the cervix, and partially encloses the perineum.

History[2]

Danish physician Lasse Hessel created it to shield partners from ejaculated semen and other bodily fluids during vaginal sex. His product first appeared in 1990 in Europe and gained the Food and Drug Administration (FDA) approval and widespread distribution in the United States the following year. There were a few different iterations of a female condom that appeared between 1920 and 1960, but they were never extensively adopted and are now largely forgotten. The spread of HIV/AIDS and the pressing need for more options in barrier methods under female control have rekindled academic interest in this area of study. In the 1980s, three groups in Europe and the United States began working on innovative designs for female condoms. These groups were "Femidom (Reality), the Bikini Condom, and Women's Choice".

Types: Only the FC1 and FC2 brands of female condoms have been approved by the FDA in the United States. There is no longer any production of the polyurethane-based female condom FC1. FC1 and FC2 have a synthetic latex option for persons who are allergic to natural rubber latex. It comes with a silicone-based lubrication already applied.

TABLE 1: Different types of contraceptives based on effectiveness.

Description	*Method examples*	*Pregnancy per 100 woman years*
Most effective	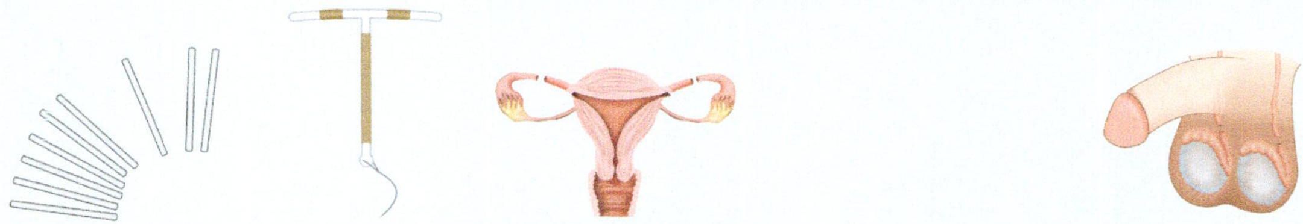 Implants, IUD, Female sterilization, Vasectomy	<2
Very effective	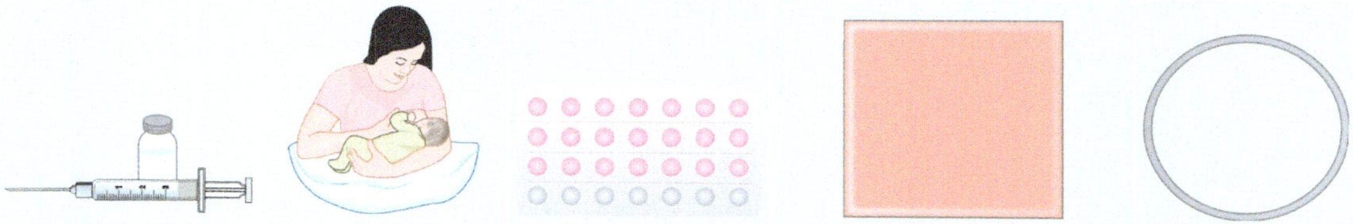 Injectables, LAM, Pills, Patch, Vaginal ring	3–9
Effective	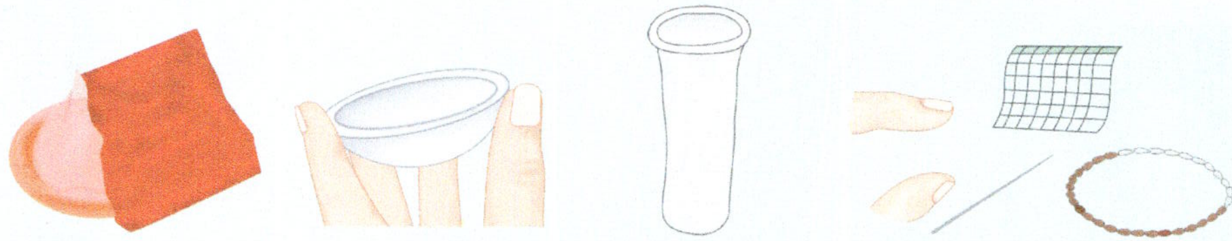 Male condom, Diaphragm, Female condom, Fertility awareness methods	10–20
Least effective	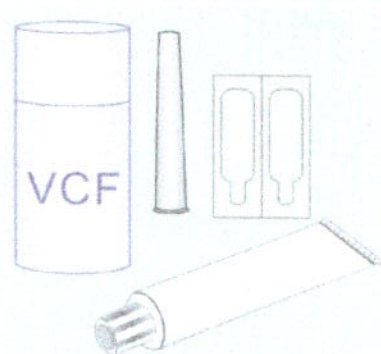 Spermicides	21–30

(IUD: intrauterine devices; LAM: lactation amenorrhea method)

Source: Hoffman BL, Schorge JO, Bradshaw KD, Halvorson LM, Schaffer JI, Corton MM., et al. Williams Gynecology 3rd edition. McGraw-Hill Education, New York, 2016.

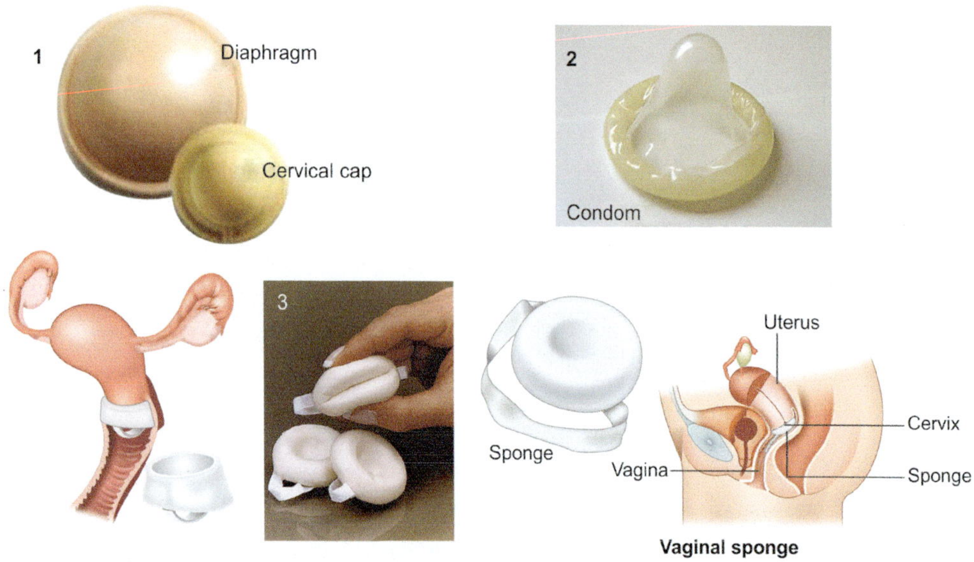

Fig. 1: Female barrier methods (1 to 3).

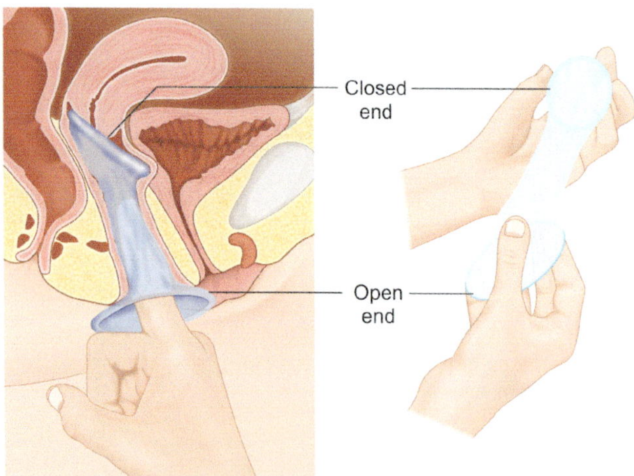

Fig. 2: Structure of a female condom.
Source: MedlinePlus [Internet]. Bethesda (MD): National Library of Medicine (US); [reviewed 2022 Oct 1]. Barrier methods of birth control-female condom; Available from: https://medlineplus.gov/ency/presentations/100107_5

In India, you can find these vaginal condoms under the brand names Femshield and Femidom structure.

Structure: Each end of the condom has a ring. The cervix is covered by the rubber material of the ring that is inserted inside the vagina. Other ring is open wide **(Fig. 2)**.

Effectiveness of female condom: "Female condoms are 95% effective when used perfectly."[3]

"British experts researching the Femidom country version validated a 1988 12-month contraceptive efficacy trial, finding a 15% failure rate among the 100 women evaluated."[4]

Medical eligibility: If they are not allergic to latex, most people can use condoms securely and successfully.

Insertion Technique

Open the package and carefully remove the condom, taking care not to rip it. You should not use your teeth to rip open the package. After locating the inner ring of the condom, hold it between your thumb and index finger. Squeeze the ring and insert it as far up the vagina as possible. Double check that the inner ring goes all the way to the bone. Keep the outer ring outside of your vaginal area. Make sure the condom is not twisted before using it. A few drops of water-based lubricant should be applied to the penis prior to initiating sexual activity and as needed during the act itself. It is important to insert the penis inside the female condom, rather than between the condom and the vaginal side. Pinch and twist the outer ring before getting up from a sexual session. After sexual contact but before getting up, squeeze and twist the outer ring to keep the semen inside. Gently yank on the condom to remove it **(Figs. 3A to J)**. One-time use only.

Disposing of female condoms: Condoms should always be thrown in the trash. A female condom should never be flushed into the toilet. It will probably clog the pipes **(Fig. 3K)**.

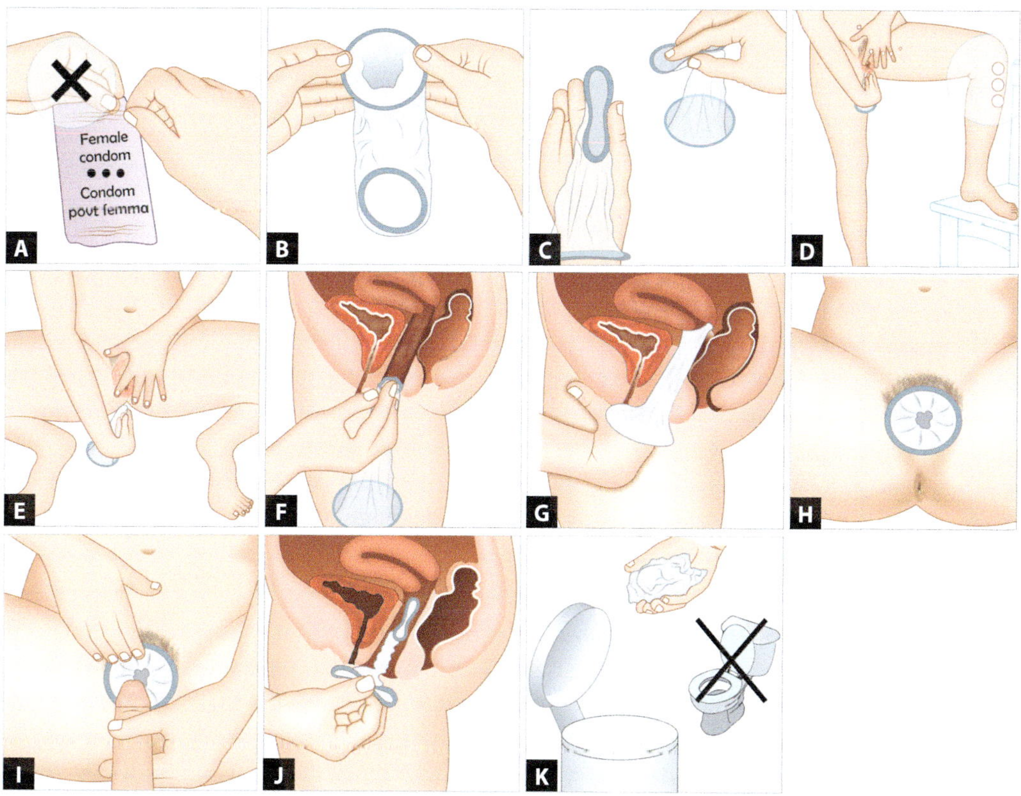

Figs. 3A to K: Insertion technique as well as disposing of female condoms. Figure (A) depicting to carefully open and remove the condom from package to prevent tearing.
Source: National Center for HIV, Viral Hepatitis, STD, and TB Prevention, Centers for Disease Control and Prevention.

Advantages

- Female condoms aid in preventing sexually transmitted infections (STIs), such as HIV, for both partners.
- They are a reliable contraceptive for preventing pregnancy when used properly.
- It is a type of contraception that you only need to use whilst doing the act.
- Can be applied to postpartum, pregnancy, or menstruation.
- There are no harmful adverse effects.
- Accessible over the counter.

Disadvantages

- Higher failure rate
- Slight possibility of toxic shock syndrome (TSS)
- Higher likelihood of urinary tract infections
- Women who have a deficient perineum, uterine prolapse, a significant cystocele, a rectocele, or a retroverted uterus should not use this product.
- Advised for one use only
- Greater cost than a male condom
- Interferes with enjoyment
- Make noise during the coitus.

Limitation: During sexual activity, sperm may occasionally enter the vagina.

This can happen if the penis touches the vagina prior to inserting a female condom, if the condom is inserted too deeply, if the penis slips between the vagina's sides, or if the condom is injured by something like jewelry sharp fingernails.

There is a chance that the condom's friction reduces the benefits of lubrication and stimulation. The use of lubrication can be helpful, but it also has the potential to make sexual action unpleasant or unsatisfying. Possible sensitivity and irritation.

Important tips:

- Avoid using jewelry or sharp fingernails to rip condoms.
- *Do not* use a male and a female condom both at the same time. They can tear as a result of friction.
- A lubricant made of petroleum, such as Vaseline, should not be used. These materials disintegrate latex.

Newer female condoms: FC2, a more recent type of female condom, is half as expensive as FC1 and is made of synthetic latex. VA feminine latex bag with a V-shaped outer frame that is prepared with a condom. Women's condoms from Path are undergoing trials.

Future Perspective of Female Condom[5]

The new female condom has the potential to increase gender equity by providing women with a product they feel comfortable purchasing and the ability to control to ensure proper use; however, future programming should address the high perceived cost of the feminine condom and women's limited decision-making power in relationships. The results also highlight the significance of demonstrating the benefits of the female condom over their male counterparts in promotional initiatives. Future social marketing methods aimed at increasing voluntary uptake should take into account the challenges discussed here.

Vaginal Diaphragm (Fig. 4)

Introduction

The diaphragm is made out of a spherical and flexible rubber dome with a range of sizes that is held in place by a metal spring around its circumference. They are included as third-tier methods in terms of effectiveness (barrier methods). It works by stopping sperm from entering the cervix.

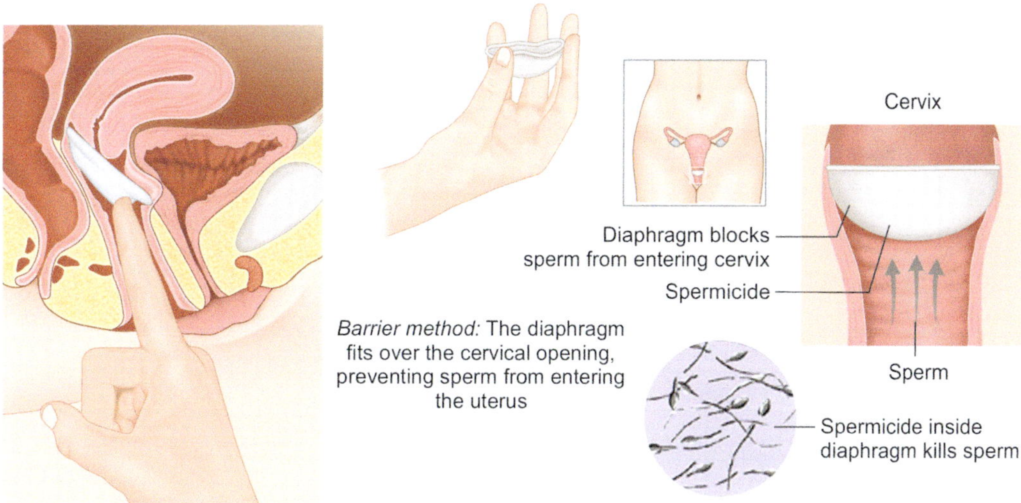

Fig. 4: Vaginal diaphragm.
Source: MedlinePlus [Internet]. Bethesda (MD): National Library of Medicine (US); [reviewed 2022 Oct 1]. Barrier methods of birth control-diaphragm. Available from: https://medlineplus.gov/ency/presentations/100107_4.

History[6]

The vaginal diaphragm, first developed in 1842, ranks among the first methods of contraception. In 1842, the diaphragm was invented by German gynecologist Dr Willhelm Mensinga. It was unquestionably popular in Europe at the turn of the century. American inventor Charles Goodyear, whose surname is synonymous with tyres, gave up on this concept in the 1850s. Goodyear was born in Connecticut. The market for such gadgets was thriving prior to the passage of the Comstock laws in the 1870s. Contraceptive methods and information were included in the list of "obscene, vulgar, and/or lascivious" things that may not be mailed. Margaret Higgins Sanger came to the rescue at this critical juncture. While visiting Holland, Sanger came across the snugly fitting spring-loaded diaphragms developed in Germany in the 1880s. After being arrested in 1916 for introducing women to these technologies, she kept spreading the word.

Structure of Diaphragm (Fig. 5)

Types: Available in three main types: (1) Flat, (2) coil, and (3) arching.

Diaphragms can have a diameter of anything from 50 mm to 105 mm (about 2-4 inches). Materials include latex and silicone. Different types of rim-mounted springs can be found in a wide variety of diaphragms.

Folding into an arc form when the edges are compressed, an arcing spring is so named. This is the most robust rim style typically offered in a diaphragm and is recommended for women of all vaginal tones. Women with mild cystocele, rectocele, or retroversion also need arcing springs, unlike other spring types. Arcing spring diaphragms are additionally less difficult to correctly install than other spring types.

As the edges of a coil spring are squeezed, the spring flattens out into an oval. Since it is not as robust as the arcing spring, this rim is only recommended for women with average or firm vaginal tones. If the diaphragm of an arcing spring causes discomfort for either

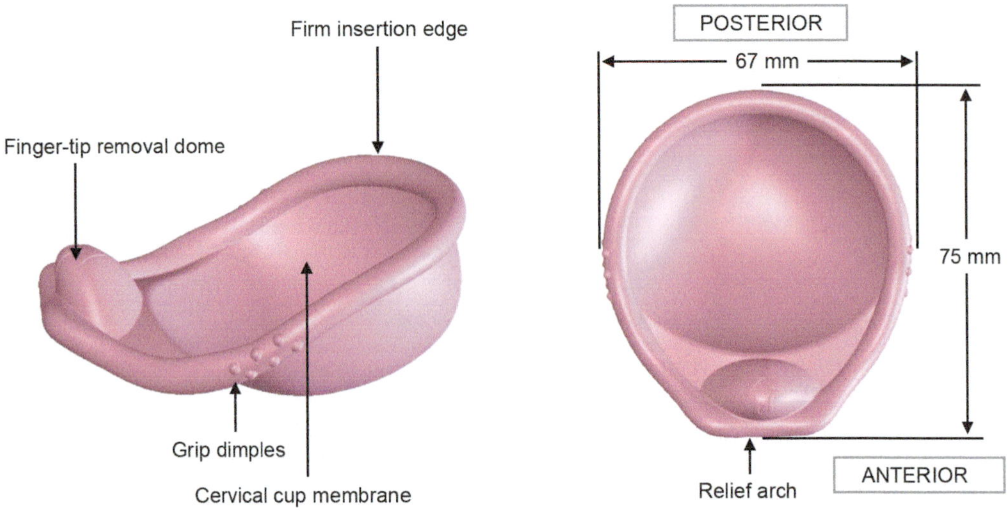

Fig. 5: Anterior and posterior structure of diaphragm.
Source: Jill L Schwartz, Susan A Ballagh, Mitchell D Creinin, Robert W Rountree, Maggie Kilbourne- Brook, Christine K Mauck, et al. SILCS diaphragm: postcoital testing of a new single-size contraceptive device, Contraception. 2008;78(3):237-44.

you or your partner, a spring may be a better option. An introducer is used to position coil springs, which are installed in a manner similar to that of arcing spring diaphragms.

Flat springs are extremely narrow iterations of traditional springs. Only women with robust vaginal tone should wear this rim style. If a woman is not confident utilizing a flat spring diaphragm, she can always resort to employing an introducer.

Effectiveness

"With regular use, the 1-year failure rate is roughly 12%, making it just moderately effective."[7]

Effectiveness is user-dependent:[8] When the diaphragm with spermicide is not used with every act of sex, the risk of pregnancy is highest. According to standard practice, there were 17 pregnancies per 100 women who used spermicide in the diaphragm during the first year. According to this, 83 out of every 100 women who use the diaphragm did not get pregnant. About 16 pregnancies were found per 100 women utilizing the diaphragm with spermicide during the first year when used appropriately with every sexual act.

Return of fertility upon cessation of diaphragmatic use: No postponement

Protection against STIs: Though it should not be relied upon to prevent STIs, it may offer some protection against

Medical eligibility: In general, anyone can use diaphragms safely and successfully as long as they are not allergic to latex, fitted no earlier than 6 weeks after giving birth or having an abortion in the second trimester, and not used for HIV protection.

*Diaphragm insertion **(Figs. 6A to D)**:*
- Select a comfortable grip by squatting, elevating one leg, sitting, or lying down.
- Put two 2 cm spermicide strips on top of the diaphragm using clean hands.

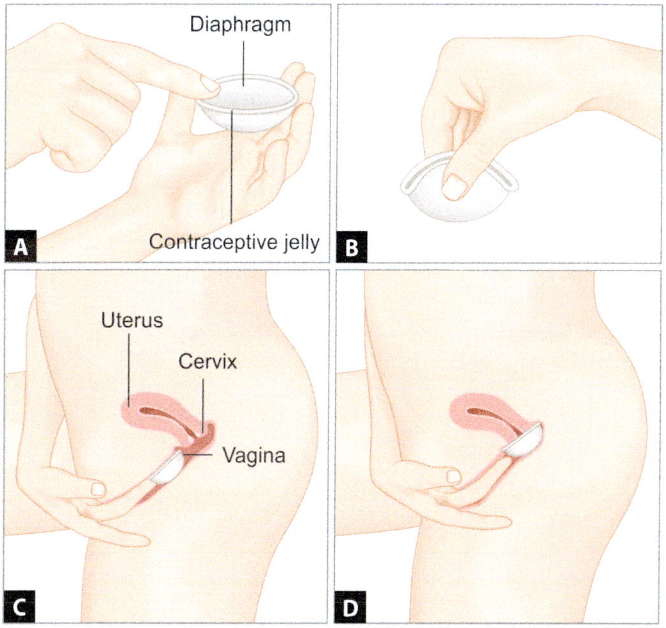

Figs. 6A to D: Diaphragm of birth control.
Source: Textbook of UP NHM community health questions.

- The diaphragm should be squeezed between your thumb and other fingers with your forefinger on top of it.
- To ensure that the diaphragm covers your cervix, slide it into your vagina and upward.
- Put your forefinger on top of the diaphragm and squeeze it between your thumb and other fingers.
- To ensure that the diaphragm covers your cervix, slide it into your vagina and upward.
- Always check to see whether your cervix is roofed; it resembles a lump and feels somewhat like the tip of your nose. If your cervix is not covered, remove the diaphragm by tugging downward on it with your finger while securing it beneath the rim or loop (if there is one), and then try again.

Instructions for usage: For use, the spermicidal agent and diaphragm are frequently inserted well before intercourse, but for maximum protection, extra spermicide is administered in the upper vagina if >2 hours have passed. Similar placement of spermicide precedes each coitus. After sexual activity, the diaphragm is not removed for at least 6 hours. The diaphragm is not left in place for longer than 24 hours because toxic shock syndrome has been linked to its use.

Advantages

- Aid in reducing pregnancy-related hazards.
- Helping to prevent certain STIs (chlamydia, gonorrhea, pelvic disease, and trichomoniasis).
- There is some defense against cervical cancer and precancer.

Disadvantages

- Initially, a doctor or other skilled individual must show proper insertion technique.

- It can only be used once the uterus has fully involuted (at least 6 weeks following delivery).
- If left in the vagina for a long time, there is a danger of TSS syndrome.
- It cannot be applied to a big cystocele or a damaged perineum.
- Additionally, it has a significant failure rate that could be decreased by the use of spermicides.

Limitation: Effective use of the diaphragm necessitates high levels of drive.

Care of diaphragm: After each usage, wash the diaphragm with mild soap and clean water, then dry it.

Correcting Misunderstandings[9]

- *Do not* interfere with the sexual experience. While some men claim to feel the diaphragms during intercourse, while most do not.
- Unable to cross the cervix.
- They cannot get lost anywhere inside the woman's body, including the uterus.
- Do not contribute to cervical cancer.

Newer Diaphragm[10]

Without the need for a provider who has been especially trained to fit the diaphragm, the one-size SILCS diaphragm has been designed to fit the majority of women. Because it is made of silicone, it is simpler to handle than traditional latex diaphragms. In 36 nations, it is registered under the name Caya. It provides comparable protection to a normal diaphragm when used with a spermicidal gel.

Cervical CAPS

Introduction

This reusable, washable, and spermicide-paired silicone barrier device surrounds the cervix to prevent the flow of sperm. Based on effectiveness, they fall within the category of third-tier procedures (barrier methods) **(Figs. 7A and B)**.

History[11]

The device, which was found in 1908 by a doctor from Vienna, is believed to have been invented in the 19th century. The 1960s saw the

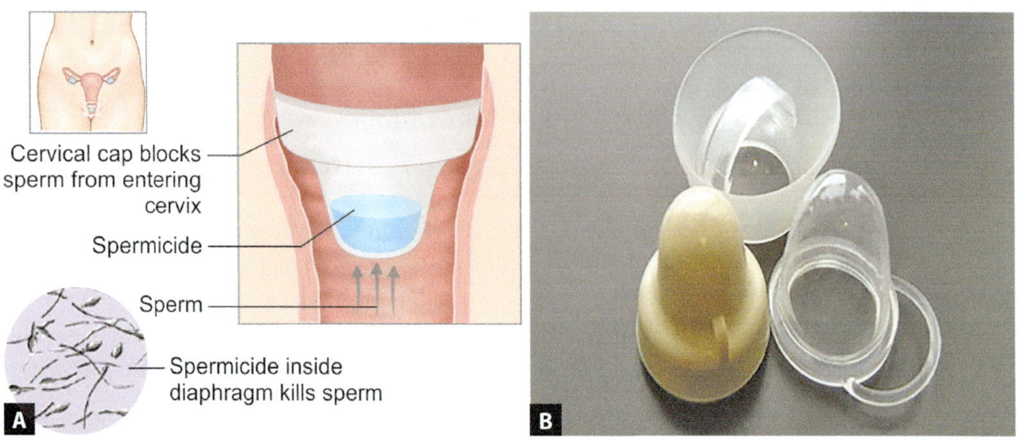

Figs. 7A and B: Cervical caps.
Source: MedlinePlus [Internet]. Bethesda (MD): National Library of Medicine (US); [reviewed 2022 Oct 1]. Barrier methods of birth control-cervical cap. Available from: https://medlineplus.gov/ency/presentations/100107_3

introduction of the IUD and oral contraceptives, which caused interest in barrier technology to wane. The US has never been the primary market for the cap; Europe has.

Structure

Cervical caps are available in 22-, 26-, and 30-mm diameters to accommodate various cervical sizes.

Effectiveness

"If a woman has never given birth, the cervical cap is far more successful. The cervical cap is 86% successful for nulligravida's. Considering the Pearl index the cap is 80.4% effective".[12]

Medical Eligibility (Table 2)

TABLE 2: Medical eligibility criteria for occlusive caps.

Category 4	None
Category 3	• History of TSS • Uterine or vaginal abnormalities • High risk of HIV • Allergy to latex • Inability of the user to insert
Category 2	• FTVD within 6–12 weeks • Parous women • Complicated valvular disease

(FTVD: full term vaginal delivery; TSS: toxic shock syndrome)
Source: https://fphandbook.org/side-effects-health-benefits-and-health-risks-1

How are They Inserted?

Fitting: A doctor selects cap size based on vaginal examination and a woman's reproductive history.

Insertion: A woman inserts it before each intercourse **(Figs. 8 A to C)**.

How do They Work?

With spermicide, they prevent pregnancy by:
- Blocking sperm from entering cervix
- Destroying sperm in the vagina

In order to be effective, they should be:
- Inserted up to *2 hours before sex*
- Left in place for at least *6 hours after sex*
- Worn for no longer than 48 hours

Advantages (Table 3)

- Reusable and reasonably priced
- Conveniently compact and portable
- There is less of a need for spermicide.
- Hormone-less
- Rarely interferes with the pleasure of having sex
- Within a 48-hour period, it is possible to engage in repeated sexual activity.
- Does not necessitate partner cooperation.

Disadvantages (Table 3)

- Demands continual use during each sexual encounter

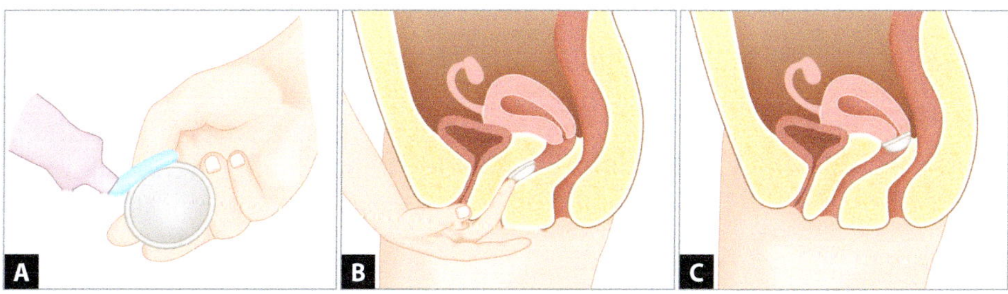

Figs. 8A to C: Techniques to insert cervical cap in the vagina. (A) Apply spermicide in the cap and its rim; (B) Fold and insert it in the vagina; (C) Make sure it covers the cervix.
Source: Textbook of UP NHM community health questions.

TABLE 3: Advantages and disadvantages of usage of cervical caps.

PROS	*CONS*
• Do not contain hormones • Reusable for up to 2 years • Work right after insertion • Do not hinder fertility	• Effectiveness ranges from 71 to 86% • Do not protect from STDs • Must be inserted before each sex • May not be suitable for all women

(STDs: sexually transmitted diseases)
Source: www.shecares.com

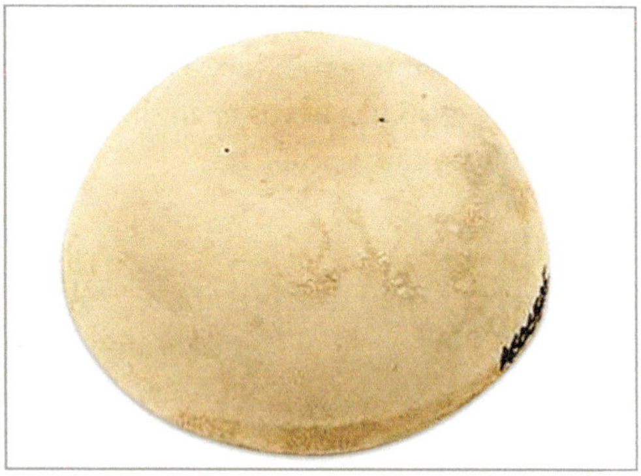

Fig. 9: Vault cap.
Source: Textbook of Clinical Obstetrics and Gynaecology, 3ed.

- Spermicide is unpleasant.
- You need a prescription.
- May increase the risk of tract infections.
- Cannot stops STDs.
- Might result in cervicitis.
- Needs to be cleaned.
- After a pregnancy, weight rise (of at least 9 kg), weight loss, an abortion, or pelvic surgery, it may be necessary to resize.
- Might become trapped within the cervix, necessitating evacuation by your healthcare provider.

Vault Cap

One type of barrier contraception is a vault cap. It rests on the cervix and blocks the sperm from entering the uterus. To conceal the cervix, it clings to the vaginal roof **(Fig. 9)**.

Evidence

- Cook LA, Nanda K, Grimes DA, Lopez LM. Diaphragm versus diaphragm with spermicides for contraception. Cochrane Database Syst Rev. 2003;(1):CD002031.
- Hassoun D. Méthodes de contraception naturelle et méthodes barrières. RPC contraception CNGOF [Natural Family Planning methods and Barrier: CNGOF Contraception Guidelines]. Gynecol Obstet Fertil Senol. 2018;46(12):873-82.
- Kuyoh MA, Toroitich-Ruto C, Grimes DA, Schulz KF, Gallo MG. Sponge versus diaphragm for contraception. Cochrane Database Syst Rev. 2002;(3):CD003172.

CONCLUSION

- Barrier methods of contraception are among the oldest techniques of pregnancy prevention.
- Mechanical barrier contraceptives are devices that provide a physical barrier between the sperm and the egg.
- Barrier methods pose a unique challenge for users as coitus-dependent contraception.
- The contraceptive efficacy of all barrier methods depends on their consistent and correct use.
- Condoms can be very effective in preventing pregnancy and STDs when used consistently and correctly.
- Barrier methods do not affect the natural hormones & milk Production.

REFERENCES

1. Hoffman BL, Schorge JO, Bradshaw KD, Halvorson LM, Schaffer JI, Corton MM., et al.

Williams Gynecology 3rd edition. McGraw-Hill Education, New York, 2016.
2. Bounds W. Female condoms. Eur J Contracept Reprod Health Care. 1997;2(2):113-6.
3. https://www.nhs.uk/conditions/contraception/female condoms/#:~:text=If%20used%20correctly%2C%20female%20condoms,UKCA%20mark%20on%20the%20packet.
4. New data found on failure rates for female condom. Rates similar to those of other barrier methods. Contracept Technol Update. 1995;16(4):54-5.
5. Gambir K, Pinchoff J, Obadeyi O, Ngo TD. Opportunities and challenges for the introduction of a new female condom among young adults in urban Zambia. Reprod Health. 2019;16(1):175.
6. https://www.reproductiveaccess.org/2013/04/a-history-the-diaphragm/
7. Wipf, Joyce (2015). Women's Health, An Issue of Medical Clinics of North America. Elsevier Health Sciences. p. 508. ISBN 9780323376082. Archived from the original on 2017-09-24
8. https://fphandbook.org/how-effective-spermicides
9. https://fphandbook.org/correcting-misunderstandings
10. https://fphandbook.org/questions-and-answers-about-spermicides-and-diaphragms
11. Gilbirds WM 2nd, Jonas HS. The cervical cap. An alternate barrier contraceptive method. Mo Med. 1982;79(4):216-8, 224.
12. Boehm D. The cervical cap: effectiveness as a contraceptive. J Nurse Midwifery. 1983;28(1):3-6.

CHAPTER 11

Male Condom

Sonali Deshpande, Apurva S Sholapure

INTRODUCTION

Condoms are considered third-tier methods (barrier methods) for male contraception due of their limited effectiveness. The condom is a simple but effective form of birth control if used correctly and frequently. Because it offers twofold protection, it has a unique position among contraceptives. It protects against sexually transmitted diseases in addition to unwanted pregnancies. Effectively preventing unwanted pregnancies requires the involvement of both sexes, and this method ensures that men are actively involved in the process. Male condoms, often made of latex rubber, are available in a variety of sizes to accommodate a wide range of sizing needs. Some condoms are lubricated, and some even incorporate spermicide **(Fig. 1)**.

HISTORY OF CONDOM

The first known usage of a condom occurred on Crete under the reign of Minos. When Pasiphae heard that her husband's semen included "scorpions and serpents" that killed his lovers, she placed a goat's bladder into her vagina to keep him away. As a form of social differentiation and bilharzia prevention, the Egyptians wore colored variations of condom-like glans caps. Animal bladders were used by the ancient Romans to shield women from sexually transmitted diseases,

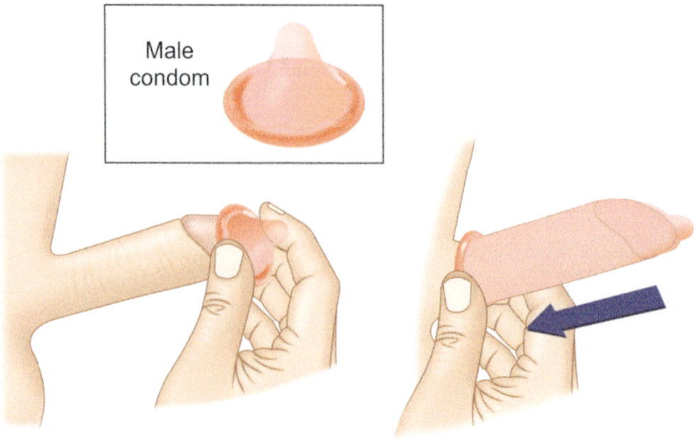

Fig. 1: Male condoms.
Source: (https://www.cdc.gov/condomeffectiveness/external-condom-use.html)

not to prevent pregnancy. Vulcanization, a procedure that softens rubber, was the basis for Charles Goodyear's development of the latex condom. Rising condom usage in the 20th and 21st centuries has been attributed to efforts to reduce the spread of the HIV virus. In this article, we will examine the history of the condom and see how a simple idea became a product that is used all over the world; in 2015, it was estimated that 18 billion condoms would be consumed.[1]

TYPE AND DISTRIBUTION

Condoms are spherical cylinders that range in length from 15 to 20 cm, in diameter from 3 to 3.5 cm, and in thickness from 0.0003 to 0.007 cm. The opposite ends are open and closed, respectively. Typically, condoms are wrapped onto the rim of the packaging and sealed with aluminum or plastic foil. The Government of India produces and provides free "Nirodh" dry condoms to its citizens. A variety of condoms, including lubricated and spermicidal kinds, are available for purchase **(Fig. 2)**.

EFFECTIVENESS OF CONDOMS

"With correct use, the failure rate is 2/100 women year as opposed to 13,100 women years with typical use".[2] In general, the failure rate is much higher during the 1st year of use. Condom effectiveness is noticeably improved by reservoir tip. Oil-based lubricants damage latex condoms, hence, the lubricant must be water-based. With every coital act, placement before penis and vagina contact, withdrawal when the penis still erects, holding the base of the condom during withdrawal, and use with spermicide are all procedures that should be taken to ensure the condom's effectiveness.

BENEFITS OF USING CONDOMS

- Avoiding unintended pregnancy
- Avoid STIs, such as HIV
- By preventing HPV transmission, assist in preventing premalignant cervical lesions
- No hormonal side effects, convenient, and safe
- Available without a prescription

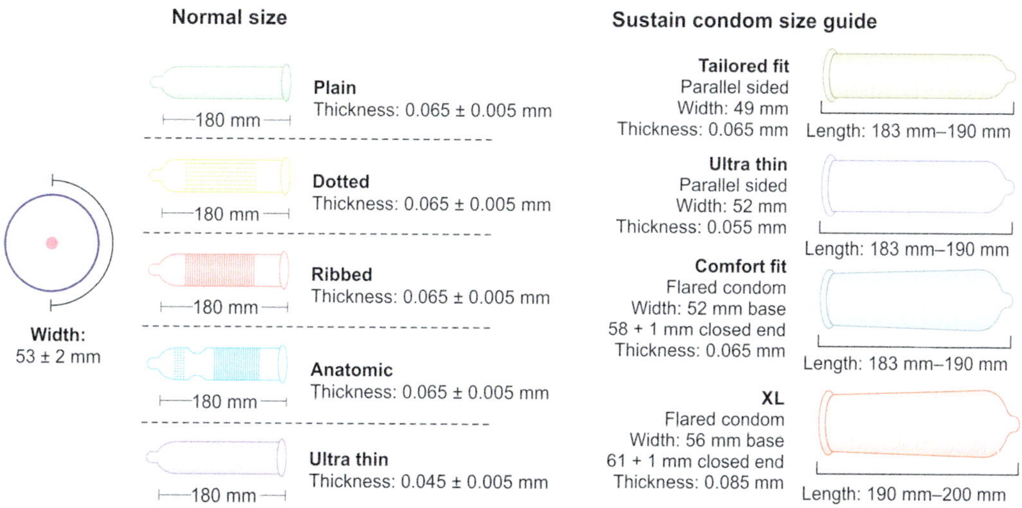
Normal size
Plain
Thickness: 0.065 ± 0.005 mm
180 mm
Dotted
Thickness: 0.065 ± 0.005 mm
180 mm
Ribbed
Thickness: 0.065 ± 0.005 mm
180 mm
Anatomic
Thickness: 0.065 ± 0.005 mm
180 mm
Ultra thin
Thickness: 0.045 ± 0.005 mm
180 mm
Width:
53 ± 2 mm
Sustain condom size guide
Tailored fit
Parallel sided
Width: 49 mm
Thickness: 0.065 mm
Length: 183 mm–190 mm
Ultra thin
Parallel sided
Width: 52 mm
Thickness: 0.055 mm
Length: 183 mm–190 mm
Comfort fit
Flared condom
Width: 52 mm base
58 + 1 mm closed end
Thickness: 0.065 mm
Length: 183 mm–190 mm
XL
Flared condom
Width: 56 mm base
61 + 1 mm closed end
Thickness: 0.085 mm
Length: 190 mm–200 mm

Fig. 2: Different types of sizes of condoms.
Source: (https://www.sciencedirect.com/science/article/abs/pii/S1521693419301774)

- Suitable for usage at any age
- Enables one to assume responsibility for preventing sickness and pregnancy.

LIMITATION

A latex allergy can cause condoms to cause irritation. Condoms made from lamb intestine are a good alternative for ladies who have an allergy to latex condoms. It appears, however, that these condoms do not protect against sexually transmitted diseases. Polyurethane condoms are hypoallergenic and highly effective at preventing sexually transmitted diseases. However, there is a greater chance of breakage and slipping than with latex condoms.

Medical eligibility: If one is not allergic to latex, one can generally use condoms securely and successfully.

DIRECTION OF USE (FIG. 3)

Verify the integrity of the condom packaging. Use caution when handling condoms from a tampered package. Condoms should never be used after their expiration date. Avoid using your teeth, nails, or anything sharp to tear open the package; instead, use your hands. You should unroll the condom and place it on the excited penis well before the tip of the condom touches the vagina, holding it so the rolled rim is facing up and away from the penis. After using a condom, you should grab the edge and place it at the base of your penis to keep it from slipping out. The person should take his penis away from the vagina without getting any semen on the vaginal opening before completely losing his erection. Make an effort to tie a knot in the condom's edge. Get rid of it by burying it or

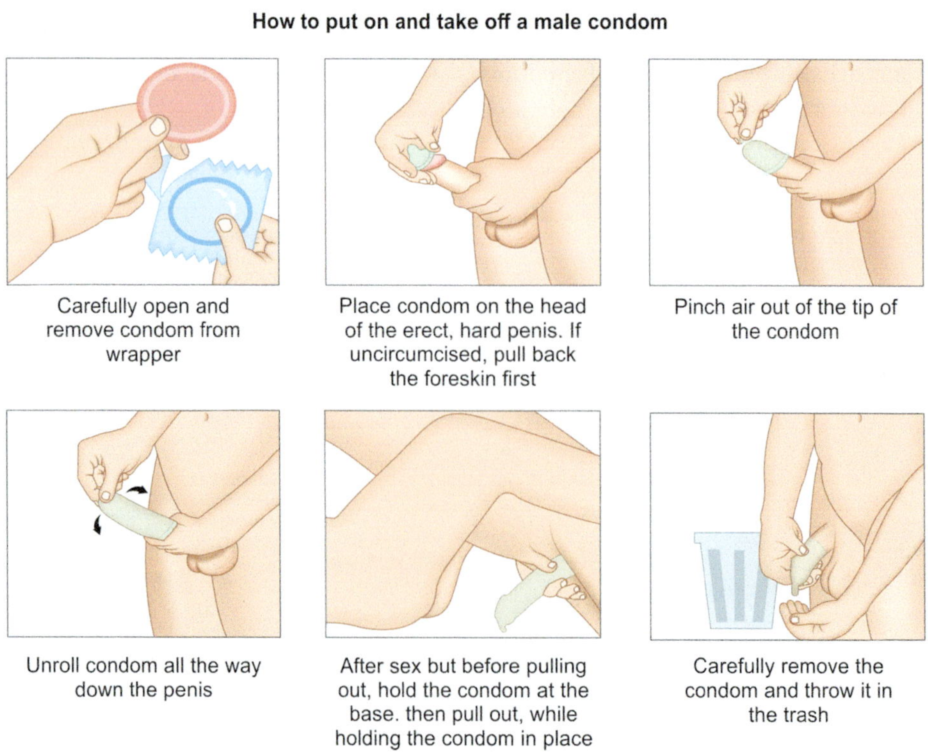

Fig. 3: Direction of condom usage.

burning it. Always use a new condom when engaging in sexual activity. Once the condom has been compromised, a spermicide should be applied to the vaginal area. If spermicides are not accessible, you can lower your risk of pregnancy and sexually transmitted infections by washing your penis and vagina with soap and water.[3]

DON'TS AND DO'S

- Do verify the expiration date on the package.
- Verify that there are no cuts.
- Do store condoms in a cool and dry environment.
- Use condoms made of latex or polyurethane.
- To stop it from breaking, use a lubricant that is silicone or water-based.
- Condoms should not be kept in wallets since the friction and heat could harm them.
- Avoid using lotion, jelly, or oil because these substances often lead to condom breaking.
- Avoid using multiple condoms at once.
- Use a different condom each time.

Reasons for using condoms: Condoms are recommended because they have no adverse effects, are readily available, are inexpensive, are portable, and may be purchased over-the-counter with no health risks.

Reasons for not using condoms: Lack of privacy in stores and societal stigma were factors in why people did not use condoms. Unpredictable male participation, decreased comfort, and decreased sexual satisfaction are the reasons condoms are not used.

FUTURE PERSPECTIVE OF CONDOMS

Graphene condoms, which are manufactured from a single layer of the material, are thinner and better at conducting heat than latex condoms. The nanolubricated condom has a covering of superhydrophilic nanoparticles (an ultra-thin layer of trapped water). The coating, made through nanofabrication, has the potential to outlast the present lubricant we use. As for other ways from the future, there are invisible condoms and ones that are powered by technology you wear. After insertion, the gel that makes up invisible condoms hardens due to body heat. They have been shown to effectively protect against HSV and HIV in laboratory studies. The barrier gives way and turns liquid after many hours have passed. The drug-treated condom is meant to assist the user keep his erection, which in turn should prevent slippage.[4,5]

KEY POINTS

- Condom use is acceptable and feasible.
- The effectiveness of condoms increases with consistent and correct use.
- The condom has dual protection role for the prevention of unwanted pregnancies as well as for the prevention of STDs.

EVIDENCE

Cochrane Library
Cochrane Database of Systematic Reviews

1. Weller SC, Davis-Beaty K. Condom effectiveness in reducing heterosexual HIV transmission. Cochrane Database Syst Rev. 2002;1:CD003255.
2. Gallo MF, Grimes DA, Lopez LM, Schulz KF. Nonlatex versus latex male condoms for contraception. Cochrane Database Syst Rev. 2006;1:CD003550.
3. Lopez LM, Otterness C, Chen M, Steiner M, Gallo MF. Behavioral interventions for improving condom use for dual protection. Cochrane Database Syst Rev. 2013;10:CD010662.

REFERENCES

1. Khan F, Mukhtar S, Dickinson IK, Sriprasad S. The story of the condom. Indian J Urol. 2013; 29(1):12-5.
2. World Health Organization. (2020). Family planning/contraception methods. [online] Available from: https://www.who.int/newsroom/fact-sheets/detail/family-planning-contraception [Last accessed November, 2022].
3. Centers for Disease Control and Prevention. (2022). Condom effectiveness: Male (External) Condom Use. [online] Available from https://www.cdc.gov/condomeffectiveness/external-condom-use.html [Last accessed November, 2022].
4. Marfatia YS, Pandya I, Mehta K. Condoms: Past, present, and future. Indian J Sex Transm Dis AIDS. 2015;36(2):133-9.
5. Hoffman BL, Schorge JO, Bradshaw KD, Halvorson LM, Schaffer JI, Corton MM., et al. Williams Gynecology 3rd edition. McGraw-Hill Education, New York, 2016.

SECTION 2

Special Situation

CHAPTER 12

Emergency Contraception

(Col) Nagaraja N

INTRODUCTION

As per a study it is estimated that 44% of the pregnancies were unintended and contributed to 55.7 million abortions between 2010 and 2014,[1] around 25.1 million abortions were unsafe and mostly happening in developing countries.[2] In India, 78% of the pregnancies are unplanned and estimated that nearly 25% of them are unwanted. Approximately 10–11 illegal abortions occur for each legal abortion and nearly 20,000 women are dying annually due to abortion-related complications which can be prevented.[3] Prevention of an unwanted pregnancy through emergency contraception will help to reduce maternal deaths due to unsafe or illegal abortions. As per the World Health Organization statement emergency contraception can prevent up to 95% of the unplanned pregnancies.[4]

Emergency contraception is a method used after unprotected sexual intercourse to prevent pregnancy, commonly called as postcoital contraception or the "morning after" treatment. "Emergency contraception" is the more accurate and appropriate name, indicating the intention before the menstrual period is missed. Emergency contraception acts primarily by preventing or delaying ovulation and by preventing fertilization. It should be counseled that it is not an abortifacient.[5] In developed countries, there is an increased incidence of high-risk sexual behavior among the adolescents along with an excellent contraception awareness varying from 61 to 93%. As per the study done in Tamil Nadu in India about awareness on emergency contraception, it is only 24.1% and education regarding emergency contraception in young adults is a very important aspect of healthcare.[6]

The idea of emergency contraception was pioneered by John Morris and Gertrude van Wagenen at Yale in the 1960s with the use of high doses of estrogen. High-dose estrogen was associated with gastrointestinal side effects. To alleviate these side effects Albert Yuzpe introduced combined oral contraceptive method with decreased the estrogen content.[5] Further progress of scientific knowledge has introduced newer methods of emergency contraception with great success and least side effects.

INDICATIONS OF EMERGENCY CONTRACEPTIVE

- Any reproductive age female with unprotected or underprotected vaginal intercourse who wishes to reduce the risk of pregnancy.
- In case of sexual assault like rape
- In case of contraceptive failure such as tear of condom, failure of coitus interruptus, and expulsion of intrauterine device (IUD).

- Incorrect use of regular contraceptive methods and at risk of unwanted pregnancy.
- After accidental/voluntary sexual act without contraceptive protection among adolescents and college girls.
- For old age couple who meet very infrequently.

METHODS OF EMERGENCY CONTRACEPTIVE

See **Flowchart 1** methods of emergency contraceptive options.

COMBINED ORAL CONTRACEPTIVE METHOD (FIG. 1)

This method of emergency contraception is known as the Yuzpe method and approved by the Food and Drug Administration (FDA) in the year 1974. The following treatment regimens have been documented:[5]

- Ovral (Contains 0.05 mg ethinyl estradiol + 0.5 mg norgestrel) l: 2 tablets stat followed by 2 tablets 12 hours later.
- Alesse (Contains 0.02 mg ethinyl estradiol + 0.1 mg levonorgestrel): 5 tablets stat followed by 5 tablets 12 hours later.
- Levlen (Contains 0.03 mg ethinyl estradiol + 0.3 mg norgestrel): 4 tablets stat followed by 4 tablets 12 hours later.

This method is more effective when they are taken at the earliest following unprotected intercourse, pills should be taken within 72 hours of intercourse, but it may be given up to 120 hours. Nausea and vomiting are common with COC regimens because of their high estrogen content. An oral antiemetic taken at least 1 hour before each dose may reduce these bothersome symptoms, a 1-hour pretreatment with either 50 mg meclizine or 10-mg metoclopramide is very effective. If vomiting occurs within 2 hours of the dose a replacement dose is to be given.[7] Failure rate of COC is about 2–3%, failure rate is lowest with high doses of ethinyl estradiol given within 72 hours (0.1%), but the side effects make this as a poor choice.[5]

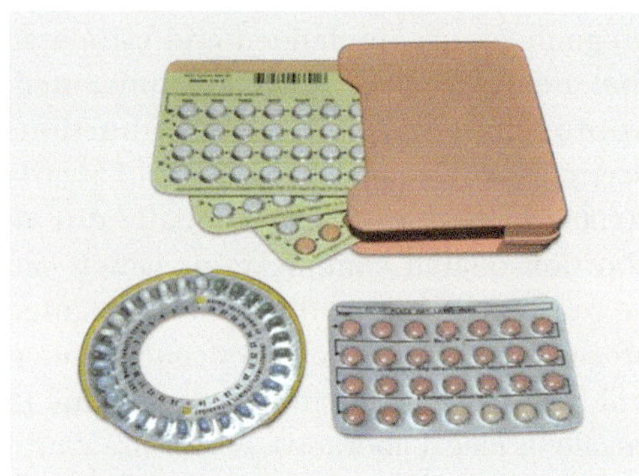

Fig. 1: Combined oral contraceptive pills.

Flowchart 1: Methods of emergency contraceptive options.

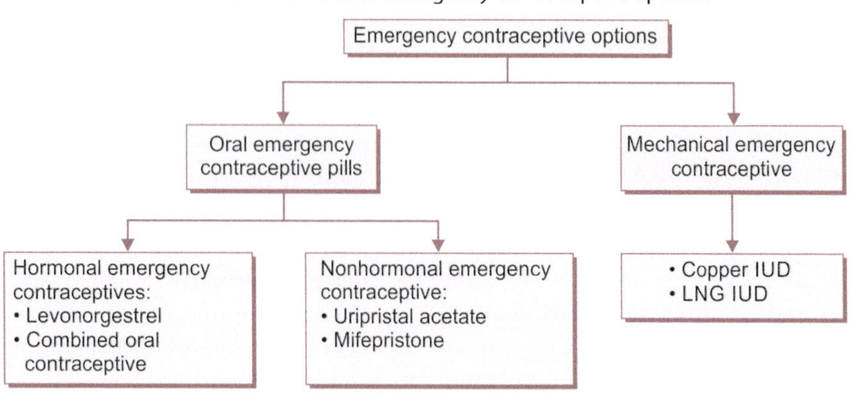

Levonorgestrel (LNG) Only Pills

It is a progestogen-based regimen most commonly used for contraception and available for emergency contraception (EC) as levonorgestrel in a dose of 0.75 mg given twice a day, 12 hours apart **(Fig. 2)**. It is a very successful and tolerated better than combination oral contraceptive method. Greater efficacy and fewer side effects make low dose levonorgestrel as the treatment of choice. In the United States, it is approved by the FDA for over-the-counter sale. The two tablets can be combined into a single dose of 1.5 mg with no loss of efficacy or increase in side effects.[5] Levonorgestrel yields a failure rate of approximately 1% with about 85% reduction in the risk of pregnancy. As per the World Health Organization study the risk of pregnancy was 60% lower with levonorgestrel only method when compared to combined oral contraceptive method with almost half the side effects.[5]

Mifepristone (Fig. 3)

It is a progesterone antagonist it acts by either delaying ovulation or impairing development of secretory endometrium. Mifepristone in a single oral dose of 600 mg is associated with markedly less nausea and vomiting than the oral contraceptives and efficacy rate is nearly 100%. In many randomized trials 10 mg mifepristone was as effective as 25, 50, or 600 mg in preventing 80–85% of expected pregnancies. It has same efficacy and side effects as levonorgestrel method with a slight decrease in efficacy when treatment was delayed to 5 days after intercourse. Because the next menstrual cycle is delayed after mifepristone, an additional method of contraception should be initiated immediately after treatment if they do not follow abstinence. It is very effective in preventing unwanted pregnancies and can induce abortions as well.[5]

Ulipristal Acetate (Fig. 4)

Ulipristal acetate has similar biologic properties like mifepristone and is approved for emergency contraception in a single

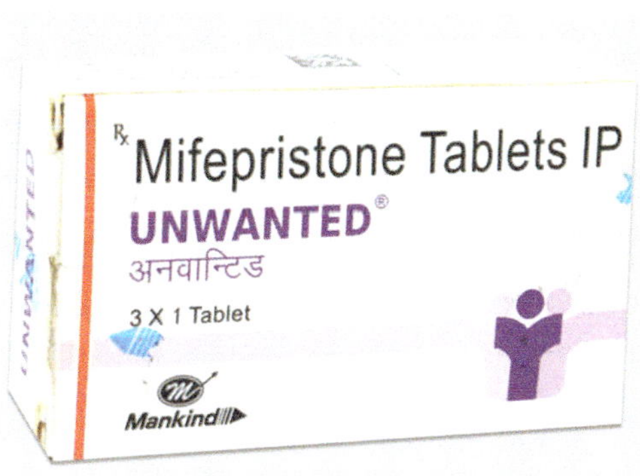

Fig. 3: Tablet mifepristone 25 mg.

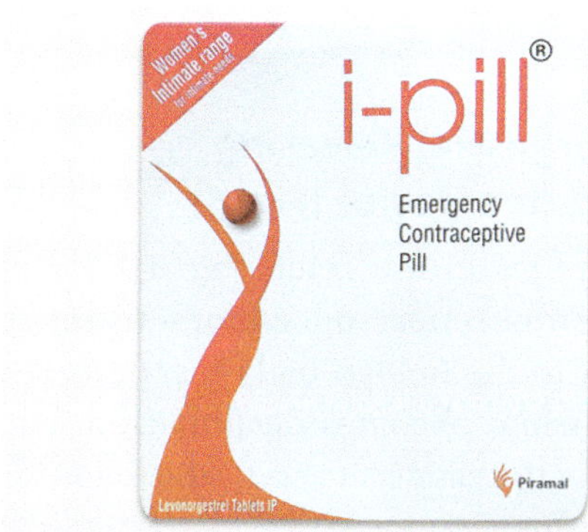

Fig. 2: Levonorgestrel emergency contraception.

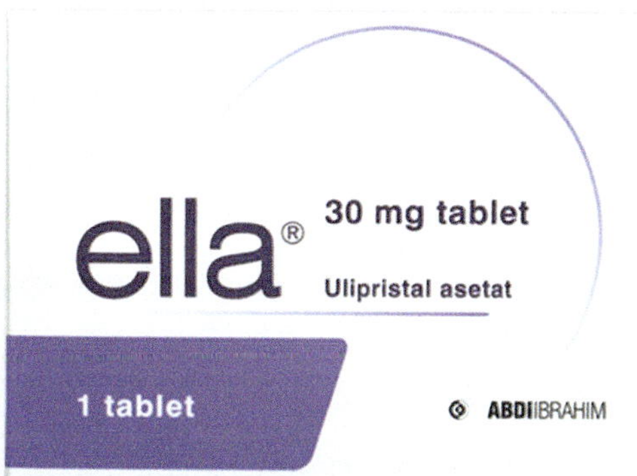

Fig. 4: Tablet ulipristal acetate.

oral dose of 30 mg. Randomized trials demonstrated that ulipristal acetate is slightly more effective than the single 1.5 mg dose of levonorgestrel when used within 72 hours or even between 72 and 120 hours after sexual intercourse. Side effects are not severe and are almost similar to levonorgestrel. Progesterone receptor modulators like ulipristal acetate and mifepristone suppress ovarian follicular growth with delay in endometrial maturation and are also associated with delay in menstruation after treatment. Ovulation may be temporarily postponed thus an immediate initiation of additional contraceptive method after treatment is very important if they do not follow abstinence.[5] After using ulipristal acetate (UPA) either barrier or pericoital contraceptives (i.e., nonhormonal contraception) can be used immediately. Women who desire progestin containing contraceptives are advised to delay start of the contraceptive for at least 5 days from the day UPA ingestion.[9] Early start of a progestin containing contraceptive could interfere with UPA function and reduce its ability to block ovulation. As per the large prospective studies, UPA is the most effective oral EC method, single cycle pregnancy rate is 1.2–1.8%.[10]

Reuse of oral emergency contraception in the same cycle: Both UPA and LNG can be used multiple times in the same menstrual cycle, although initiation of a proven contraceptive method is preferred. Oral LNG 1.5 mg has been tested as an as-needed contraceptive for women with <6 episodes of intercourse per month. Study conducted among 321 enrolees, there were 142 women years of use and the typical use pregnancy rate was 7.1 per 100 women years. More than 80% of users had frequent bleeding episodes, despite this 90% of the participants were ready to use this method again.[8,9]

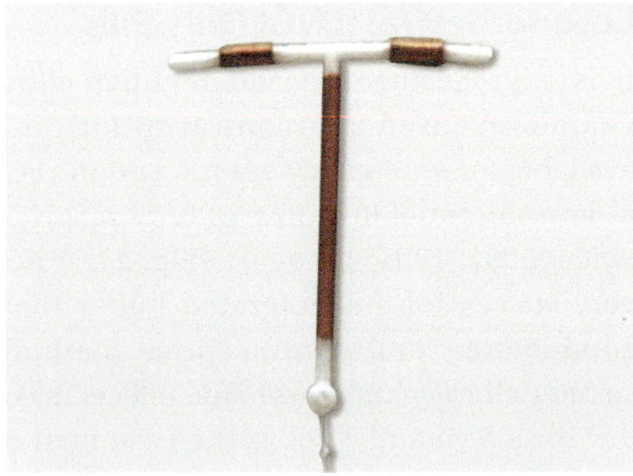

Fig. 5: Intrauterine copper devices (380A).

Copper Intrauterine Device (Fig. 5)

Copper intrauterine device (CU-T IUD) is the most effective option for emergency contraception and has been used as EC for >35 years. CU-T IUD can be used up to 5 days after an unprotected intercourse. It is effective as soon as it is inserted and gives immediate protection and also for subsequent acts. It can be used up to 3–10 years subsequently with a very low failure rate of 0.1%.[5] The copper IUD releases free copper and copper salts that have both a biochemical and morphologic impact on the endometrium, enhancing prostaglandin production, producing cytotoxic cytokine peptides, inhibiting endometrial enzymes, endometrial receptivity is also inhibited. An additional spermicidal effect may take place in the cervical mucus.[10]

Levonorgestrel Releasing Intrauterine Device (Fig. 6)

This progesterone-releasing IUD has progesterone effect on endometrium in addition to the foreign body reaction. The endometrium becomes decidualized with atrophy of the glands. It acts by the following mechanisms:

- Inhibition of implantation

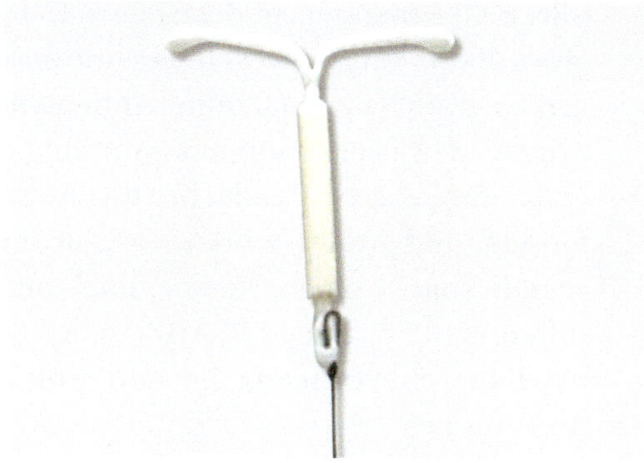

Fig. 6: Levonorgestrel releasing intrauterine system (LNG IUS).

- Thickens the cervical mucus, creating a barrier to sperm penetration
- Inhibition of sperm capacitation, penetration, and survival.

The levonorgestrel intrauterine system (IUS) produces serum concentrations of the progestin about half those of norplant so that ovarian follicular development and ovulation are also partially inhibited, after the 1st year cycles are ovulatory in 50–75% of women regardless of their bleeding patterns.[10]

Both the copper T-380A and LNG-52 mg IUD do provide EC and ongoing contraception which would not require backup contraception or abstinence. This simple approach provides the highest efficacy for both EC and contraception. A study of 518 individuals who were given either the TCu308A or LNG-52 IUDs reported that 64% resumed penile-vaginal intercourse within 7 days of IUD insertion but only 16% used a form of back-up contraception and no pregnancies occurred in either group.[9] Selection of IUD type among EC users should depend upon user preferences and the unique characteristics of each IUD. Those who prefer to avoid hormones and maintain a regular menstrual cycle mostly prefer copper IUD and whoever prefers less or no menstrual bleeding and cramping with tolerance for potential amenorrhea may prefer LNG-IUS.

Intrauterine devices have significant advantages over oral EC methods as there are very few contraindications to IUD-EC use. Main advantages of IUDs for EC are extended timing of insertion, continuing contraception, and good efficacy. Studies have reported zero pregnancies among participants reporting UPI >5 days prior to copper TCu380A IUD placement. This same dataset reported one pregnancy among 187 LNG 52 mg IUD users with UPI 6–14 days prior to IUD placement (0.5%, 95% CI: 0.01–2.9%). Society of Obstetricians and Gynaecologists of Canada advised IUD use within 7 days of UPI, and World Health Organization also says that the copper TCu380A IUD can be inserted beyond 5 days from UPI.[9] The common disadvantage being concern about pelvic inflammatory diseases following CU-T IUD insertion and, hence, it is contraindicated in women who currently known to have PID, purulent cervicitis, chlamydia, or gonorrhea infection.

SEXUAL ASSAULT AND EMERGENCY CONTRACEPTION

In cases of sexual assault emergency contraception should be offered. The Royal College of Obstetricians and Gynaecologists Faculty of Sexual and Reproductive Healthcare recommend offering the copper TCu380A intrauterine device (IUD), the most effective method of EC, to everyone at risk of pregnancy after a sexual assault. Ideally, this should immediately follow forensic examination for specimen collection.[9] Emergency oral contraceptives are also a good option for EC following sexual assault.

Impact of Body Weight

Body weight does not impact the efficacy of the copper TCu380A IUD, which in part contributes to its overall high efficacy.

Emergency contraceptive efficacy of both UPA and LNG appears to decrease with increasing body mass index (BMI) for both overweight (BMI: 25–29.9 kg/m) and obese (BMI ≥30 kg/m) individuals. A study comparing serum LNG levels in five women with normal BMI (18–24.9 kg/m) versus five obese women (BMI ≥30 kg/m) reported that, after an oral dose of 1.5 mg LNG, obese women had LNG serum levels one-half those of the controls.[11] When the oral LNG dose was doubled to 3 mg the serum level in obese women reached the level of the 1.5 mg control women. A different study that compared serum levels of LNG and UPA in 16 normal and obese women reported that obese participants had LNG levels one-half of the normal BMI participants, while UPA levels did not differ between the groups.[12]

SIDE EFFECTS OF EMERGENCY CONTRACEPTIVE

Emergency contraceptive has shown good safety profile and there are no serious or morbid complications. Emergency contraceptive may cause some side effects that are typically mild and last for short duration like:

- *Change in menstrual cycle pattern:* There may be change in menstrual cycle that follows the use of emergency contraceptive pills. These changes are due to the hormonal imbalance may cause spotting after taking pills.
- *Abnormal or irregular uterine bleeding:* Intrauterine device may cause change in bleeding pattern and sometimes heavy menstrual bleeding or intermenstrual bleeding.
- *Nausea and vomiting:* It is observed more in women who took Yuzpe regimen. Nausea does not last for >24 hours and it is less if pills are taken at bedtime. If vomiting takes place within 2 hours of pills intake then repeat dose needs to be given. If vomiting is severe then same dose can be given by vaginal route. Antiemetic drugs can be used to suppress vomiting.
- *Other side effects:* Headache, dizziness, fatigue, and breast tenderness can be seen in some women. Nonsteroidal anti-inflammatory drugs (NSAIDs) may be used to relieve headache and breast tenderness.

BENEFITS OF EMERGENCY CONTRACEPTIVE[13]

- Safe and effective
- Easy to use and widely available
- Can be taken at any time during the cycle
- Physical examination is not required
- It is available without a prescription from registered medical practitioner
- Can be given to women in whom use of hormonal contraceptive are contraindicated.
- Can be used as many times as needed; although not substitute for regular contraceptive.
- There are no serious medical complications.
- Doses of hormone are relatively small.
- Short exposure does not have any metabolic effects.
- Not associated with any fetal malformation or congenital anomalies
- Does not increase risk of ectopic pregnancy.

SAFETY AND CONTRAINDICATIONS

Emergency contraceptive pills are not very dangerous under any known circumstances. Recognized contraindications for combined oral contraceptive pills do not apply to emergency contraceptive pills. Women with history of cardiovascular diseases, thromboembolic disease, chronic liver disease, migraine, angina and breastfeeding women may use LNG pills.[14] Uripristal acetate may be avoided in breastfeeding women. If used, then women may be advised to stop breastfeeding for 1 week following use.[15] IUDs are contraindicated in women known to have PID, active gonorrhea and chlamydia infection, purulent cervicitis, and women with high risk for STD.[14]

CONCLUSION

Emergency contraceptive is a safe and effective method of contraception preventing 75–99% unwanted or unintended pregnancies and helps in reducing the risk of unsafe and illegal abortions. It is proven to be safe, convenient, and very effective for one-time protection from unwanted or unintended pregnancy following unprotected intercourse. Patients should be encouraged to use regular effective contraceptive method after start of periods. It is the responsibility of clinician to educate patient about emergency contraceptive option along with the counseling for regular contraception. Patients should be explained about available methods and offer the most suitable emergency contraceptive (EC) with a great emphasis on intrauterine copper device as it is the most effective option and it can function as a regular contraception for subsequent sexual act. EC is both a preventive and therapeutic strategy toward women healthcare, as it can avoid unintended and accidental pregnancies. It helps in the improving countries biostatistics like maternal mortality and family planning services with a great contribution toward progress of the country.

REFERENCES

1. Bearak J, Popinchalk A, Alkema L, Sedgh G. Global, regional, and sub regional trends in unintended pregnancy and its outcomes from 1990 to 2014: estimates from a Bayesian hierarchical model. Lancet Glob Health. 2018;6(4):e380-9.
2. Ganatra B, Gerdts C, Rossier C, Johnson BR Jr, Tunçalp Ö, Assifi A, et al. Global, regional, and sub-regional classification of abortions by safety, 2010-14: estimates from a Bayesian hierarchical model. Lancet. 2017;390(10110): 2372-81.
3. Arora P, Bajpai RC, Srivastava R. Emergency contraception: a study to assess knowledge, attitude and practices among female college students in Delhi. Natl J Community Med. 2013;4(2):282-5.
4. World Health Organization. (2018). Emergency contraception. Fact sheet, 2018, February. [online] Available from: https://www.who.int/news-room/fact-sheets/detail/emergencycontraception [Last accessed November, 2022].
5. Taylor HS, Pal L, Seli E. Speroff's Clinical Gynecologic Endocrinology and Infertility, 9th Edition. Netherlands: Wolters Kluwer; 2020. pp. 2314-20.
6. Davis P, Sarasveni M, Krishnan J, Bhat LD, Kodali NK. Knowledge and attitudes about the use of emergency contraception among college students in Tamil Nadu, India. J Egypt Pub Health Assoc. 2020;95:1-2.
7. Hoffman BL, Schorge JO, Bradshaw KD, Halvorson LM, Schaffer JI, Corton MM. Williams Gynecology, 3rd Edition. United States: McGraw-Hill Education; 2016. p. 132.
8. Thompson I, Sanders JN, Schwarz EB, Boraas C, Turok DK. Copper intrauterine device placement 6-14 days after unprotected sex. Contraception. 2019;100:219.
9. Turok D, Schreiber CA, Eckler K. Emergency contraception. UpToDate. 2022:5-13.
10. Taylor HS, Pal L, Seli E. Speroff's Clinical Gynecologic Endocrinology And Infertility, 9th Edition. Netherlands: Wolters Kluwer; 2020. p. 2437.
11. Edelman AB, Cherala G, Blue SW, Erikson DW, Jensen JT. Impact of obesity on the pharmacokinetics of levonorgestrel-based emergency contraception: single and double dosing. Contraception. 2016;94:52.

12. Praditpan P, Hamouie A, Basaraba CN, Nandakumar R, Cremers S, Davis AR, et al. Pharmacokinetics of levonorgestrel and ulipristal acetate emergency contraception in women with normal and obese body mass index. Contraception. 2017;95:464.
13. Guidelines for administration of emergency contraceptive pills by health care provider by Family Planning Division, Ministry of Health and Family Welfare GOI, Nov 2008.
14. World Health Organization. Medical eligibility criteria for contraceptive use. 2010.
15. Faculty of Sexual and Reproductive Health-care, Royal College of Obstetricians and Gynaecologists. Use of ulipristal acetate (ellaOne(R)) in breastfeeding women, update from the Clinical Effectiveness Unit. 2013.

CHAPTER 13

Medicolegal Aspects of Tubal Sterilization and Vasectomy

Sudesh Doshi

INTRODUCTION

India was the first country in the world to have launched a "National Program for Family Planning" in 1952. Since then "Family Planning Program" has undergone transformation in terms of policy and actual program implementation. In initial days, it was restricted to female and male sterilization. Further, it was expanded to temporary methods such as intrauterine contraceptive devices, oral contraceptive pills, and injectables. In initial days, various incentives were offered to service providers and beneficiaries.

Vasectomy failed into disrepute due to its misuse and forceful implementation during national emergency in 1975.

In spite of various efforts by Government of India and various State Governments vasectomy has not been able become a popular choice. The reasons being:

- Patriarchal mindset of Indian population where responsibility of bearing or not bearing a child rests with females.
- Deep rooted misbelief that vasectomy will damage one's sexual powers and capacity to do daily strenuous work.
- More number of female workers in family planning program to whom male population is not available for counseling.

In 1977, Government of India redesignated "National Family Program" as "National Family Welfare Program".

In year 2013–14, 38% of women in reproductive age group in India that is almost 41 lacs chose and underwent tubectomy. Thus, tubal ligation remains the most popular method of contraception.

Various guidelines have been published by Union government as well as State governments regarding eligibility and provision of service providers, beneficiaries, facilities since 1989 and revised periodically.

Mishaps including deaths keep on occurring as a result of tubectomy operation especially in camps in spite of all regulations and guidelines. For this government has restricted the number of patients undergoing sterilization to <30/day/surgeon.

Following are taken from reference manual for sterilization published by the Ministry of Health and Family Welfare in 2014.

WHO ARE ELIGIBLE TO PERFORM STERILIZATION PROCEDURE?

Those who are empaneled.

- *For female minilap sterilization:* Postgraduate degree or diploma holder in obstetrics and gynecology, MBBS who have received training in minilap and specialists in other surgical fields.
- *For laparoscopic sterilization:* Postgraduate degree or diploma holder in obstetrics and gynecology, MBBS who

have received training in minilap further training in laparoscopic sterilization and specialists in other surgical fields.

Male: Conventional vasectomy and no scalpel vasectomy, a person who is MBBS and above and trained in respective surgical techniques.

A separate list for minilap, laparoscopic tubectomy, conventional and no scalpel vasectomy providers is to be maintained by the state.

- Only empaneled doctors are entitled to carry out sterilization operations in public and accredited private/NGO facilities. The list of empaneled doctors to be maintained by state and revised 3 monthly.

  Empaneled doctors can operate all over India.
- Doctors who are already performing sterilization operation in the public should be empaneled by states.

CORRECT TIME TO PERFORM FEMALE STERILIZATION

Women Menstruating Regularly Cycles

- Any time within 7 days after the start of her menstrual bleeding.
- Any time of menstrual cycle, if it is reasonably certain that she is not pregnant.

Women Already using Some Methods from Another Method

- *If she is taking contraceptive pills:* To be done any time but she can continue the pill until the pack is finished to maintain her regular cycle.
- If she has cut in situ can done anytime, with removal of cut at the same time.

Women with No Monthly Menstrual Bleeding

If it is reasonably certain she is not pregnant. Can be done any time.

Puerperal Women

- Within 7 days after giving birth when only postpartum minilap tubectomy can be performed.
- Interval sterilization: If it is reasonably certain she is not pregnant any time 6 weeks or more after childbirth.

After MTP can be done within 7 days post MTP or Concurrently with surgical MTP.

The tubectomy should be done after next menstrual cycle if she has availed medical method of abortion.

Laparoscopic tubal occlusion procedure can be performed only in MTPs up to 12 weeks of gestation.

After uncomplicated abortion or miscarriage: Within 7 days.

After using emergency contraceptive pills (ECPs): Within 7 days after the start of her next monthly bleeding or any other time if it is reasonably certain she is not pregnant.

A woman can have the female sterilization procedure any time she wants, if there is no medical reason to delay and if it is reasonably certain that she is not pregnant.

PRESURGERY COUNSELING AND INFORMED CONSENT

What Is Counseling?

Oxford dictionary defines counseling as:

"The provision of professional guidance and assistance in resolving personal or psychological problems".

In family planning, it facilitates and enables clients to make well informed, well considered, and voluntary decisions about fertility and to choose a contraceptive method.

It is a two-way process of communication in which the service provider understands clients' perceptions, attitudes, values, beliefs, family planning needs and preferences and accordingly guides him/her toward decision making. It should be nonjudgmental.

During the process of counseling, privacy (auditory and visual) and confidentiality should be maintained.

Client's lack of information about sterilization and its effect which is further compounded by misconceptions and concerns should be dispelled by providing correct information.

Counseling has two parts general counseling and method-specific counseling.

Counseling (General)

It should be done for all the potential beneficiaries services. The general counseling provides informed choice clients to enable them to take a decision regarding the type of contraceptive method to be used.

Counseling (Method Specific)

- In this all the pros and cons related to that specific methods should be informed to potential beneficiary.
- Use of simplified schematic diagrams can be helpful in counseling about sterilization.

The following steps should be ensured before the potential beneficiary signs the consent form:

- Wherever required potential beneficiary should be counseled in the language they understand.
- Information of all the available methods of family planning and procedures should be understood by the potential beneficiary.
- It should be understood by the potential beneficiary what may happen before, during, and after the surgery, its side effects and potential complications.
- Beneficiary should make informed decision for sterilization voluntarily.
- Beneficiary should understand the following features of the sterilization procedure.
    - The sterilization procedure is a permanent surgical procedure.
    - It is a surgical procedure in which further management may be required in cases of complications, including failure.
    - Sexual pleasure, ability, or performance is not affected by undergoing sterilization.
    - The beneficiary's strength or ability to perform normal day-to-day functions is not affected.
    - Sterilization gives no protection against sexually transmitted infections (STIs), reproductive tract infections (RTIs), and human immunodeficiency virus (HIV)/acquired immunodeficiency syndrome (AIDS).
    - It is potentially reversible but the reversal involves major surgery and the success of which cannot be guaranteed.
    - There is a redressal mechanism available in the form of an indemnity coverage in the unlikely event of any complication/failure/death.

Follow-up Counseling

The information provided after the procedure is reinforced. Service providers need to listen attentively and be prepared to answer questions. The potential beneficiary may have and address problems she has experienced after undergoing the procedure. This helps the client to cope with common problems or side effects. Advise client to return to the facility if there is any missed period/ suspected pregnancy within 2 weeks to rule out pregnancy.

Informed Consent and Informed Choice

The concepts of informed consent and informed choice are quite related but different in their intent. The informed choice has a purpose to ensure that all clients after getting full information about all available options, choose the best option/s for their healthcare needs.

Informed consent means that a client understands the surgical procedure and other options and then decides to receive the care.

For sterilization, the consent of the partner is not required; however, the partner should be encouraged to come for counseling.

Documentation of Informed Consent

Must always sign or put her thumb impression on the consent from for authorization for the sterilization procedure to be performed.

In case of thumb impression, a signature of a witness (any person not associated with the service facility and chosen by the client is a must.

Consent for sterilization should not be obtained when physical or emotional factors may compromise a client's ability to make a carefully considered decision about contraception.

Proforma for Consent for Strelization

I, *Smt/Shri .... (client) hereby give consent for my sterilization operation. I am ever married. My age is .... years and my husband/wife's age is ...... years. I have .... (Nos.) male and ...... (Nos.) female living children. The age of my youngest living child is .... years.*

a. I have decided to undergo the sterilization/re-sterilization operation on my own without any outside pressure, inducement or force. I declare that I/my spouse have/has not been sterilized previously *(not applicable in case of re-sterilization).*
b. I am aware that other methods of contraception are available to me. I know that for all practical purposes this operation is permanent and I also know that there are still some chances of failure of the operation for which the operating doctor and health facility will not be held responsible by me or by my relatives or any other person whomsoever.
c. I am aware that I am undergoing an operation, which carries an element of risk.
d. The eligibility criteria for the operation have been explained to me and I affirm that I am eligible to undergo the operation according to the criteria.
e. I agree to undergo the operation under any type of anesthesia, which the doctor/health facility thinks suitable for me and to be given other medicines as considered appropriate by the doctor/ health facility concerned. I also give consent for any additional life-saving procedure, if required.
f. I agree to come for follow-up visits to the Hospital/Institution/Doctor/health facility as instructed, failing which I shall be responsible for the consequences, if any.
g. If, after the sterilization operation, I experience a missed menstrual cycle, then I shall report within 2 weeks of the missed menstrual cycle to the doctor/health facility and may avail of the facility to get an MTP done free of cost. I shall be responsible for the consequences, if any.

h. I understand that vasectomy does not result in immediate sterilization. *I agree to come for semen examination *3 months after the operation* to confirm the success of sterilization surgery (Azoospermia) failing which I shall be responsible for the consequences, if any. (**Applicable for male sterilization cases*).

i. *In case of complications, failures, and the unlikely event of death attributable to sterilization, I/my spouse and dependent unmarried children will accept the compensation as per the existing provisions of the Government of India "Family Planning Indemnity Scheme" as full and final settlement and will not be entitled to claim any other compensation including compensation for upbringing of the child, if any, born on account of failure of sterilization, over and above the one offered, from any court of law in this regard.*

I have read the above information or the above information has been read out and explained to me in my own language and that this form has the authority of a legal document.

I am aware that I have the option of deciding against the sterilization procedure at any time without sacrificing my rights to other reproductive health services.

Signature or Thumb Impression of the Client

Date: ....

Name of client: ....

Signature of Witness (Clients side): ....

Full Name: ....

I am aware that client is ever married and has one living child over 1 year of age.

Signature of ASHA/Counselor/Motivator: ....

Full Name: ....

Full Address ....

I certify that I have satisfied myself that:

a. Shri/Smt. .... is within the eligible age-group and is medically fit for the sterilization operation.

b. I have explained all clauses to the client and that this form has the authority of a legal document.

c. I have filled the medical record-cum-checklist and followed the standards for sterilization procedures laid down by the Government of India.

HOW TO DOCUMENT DENIAL OF STERILIZATION

A client who is not fit for sterilization should be counseled and offered another method of contraception. The documentation of reason for denial of sterilization must be done in the prescribed consent form given below. When an evaluation of potential beneficiary indicates sterilization to be unsuitable for her either on medical or non-medical grounds, the beneficiary record should specify the reasons (e.g., the medical/surgical condition, not sure of her choice, etc.). Then, the provider should also be described the action taken (e.g., referral, treatment, etc.). The records for the same should be kept at the service facility where the potential beneficiary was evaluated, and the sterilization found unsuitable for her.

Denial of Sterilization

I certify that Shri/Smt .... is not a suitable client for sterilization/re-sterilization for the following reasons:

1. ....
....
....
2. ....
....
....

He/She has been advised the following alternative methods of contraception.

1. ....
....
....
2. ....
....
....

Following are eligibility criteria for beneficiaries undergoing female sterilization:

(Self-declaration by the client will be the basis for compiling this information. No eligible client should be denied female sterilization service).

- Clients should be ever-married.
- Female clients should be below the age of 49 years and above the age of 22 years.
- The couple should have at least one child, who is above 1 year old, unless the sterilization is medically indicated.
- Clients or their spouses/partners must not have undergone sterilization in the past (not applicable in cases of failure of previous sterilization).
- Clients must be in a sound state of mind, so as to understand the full implications of sterilization.
- Mentally ill clients must be certified by a psychiatrist and a statement should be given by the legal guardian/spouse regarding the soundness of the client's state of mind.
- A relevant medical history, physical examination, and laboratory investigations need to be completed to ascertain eligibility for surgery.

Client assessment for eligibility to undergo female sterilization is a key factor in minimizing risk of complications and ensuring quality of service delivery. No medical conditions prevent a woman from undergoing female sterilization but may limit when, where, or how the female sterilization procedure should be performed.

Accept (A): There is no medical reason to deny the method to a person with this condition or in this circumstance. The procedure can be performed in most clinical settings.

Caution (C): The method is normally provided in a routine setting but with extra preparation and precautions as required.

History of ischemic heart disease, stroke, history of cerebrovascular accident, obesity, previous abdominal or pelvic surgery, uncomplicated heart disease, controlled BP (140–159/90–99), PID without subsequent pregnancy, hypothyroidism, epilepsy, history of DVT or pulmonary embolism, uncomplicated diabetes, uterine fibroids, epilepsy, current breast cancer depressive disorder, kidney disease, and mild cirrhosis.

Delay (D): Provision of the method should be delayed or postponed. These conditions need to be evaluated, treated, and resolved before female sterilization can be performed. Alternatively, temporary methods of contraception should be provided.

8–42 days postpartum, current pregnancy, abdominal skin infections, severe iron-deficiency anemia (hemoglobin <7 gm/dL current DVT/PE, major surgery with prolonged immobilization, current purulent cervicitis, chlamydia, gonorrhea unexplained vaginal bleeding, large collection of blood in uterus, pregnancy with severe preeclampsia or eclampsia.

Special (S): Certain women have conditions that make operation difficult or increase the risks. The procedure should be undertaken in a setting with an equipment needed to provide general anesthesia. Experienced surgeon and staff, and other back-up medical support. The capacity to decide on the most appropriate procedure and anesthesia support is also needed. Alternatively, temporary methods of contraception should be provided if referral is required or there is otherwise any delay.

Conditions that increase chances of heart disease or stroke, i.e., older age, smoking, high BP or diabetes, coagulation disorders, blood pressure >160/100 mm Hg, complicated heart disease, chronic lung diseases (asthma or emphysema), postpartum or postabortion complications, (infection, hemorrhage, and trauma,) diabetes >20 years with organ damage, endometriosis, pelvic tuberculosis, fixed uterus due to previous surgery or infection, postpartum or postabortion uterine rupture or perforation.

Current ischemic heart disease, abdominal wall or umbilical hernia, liver tumors, lung disease such as pneumonia, systemic infection, AIDS, hyperthyroidism, severe cirrhosis of liver, uncontrolled diabetes, malignant trophoblastic disease, HIV, cancers of the genital tract, current gall-bladder disease, thalassemia, and sickle-cell disease.

Offer the client another contraceptive method till the procedure can be performed.

FEMALE STERILIZATION IN WOMEN WITH HIV/AIDS

No woman should be denied female sterilization based on their HIV status.

Women who are living with HIV, have AIDS, or are on antiretroviral (ARV) therapy can safely undergo female sterilization. The procedure is done as in other clients, ensuring universal precautions.

These women should be counseled to use condoms in addition to undergo female sterilization to help to prevent transmission of HIV and other STIs (dual protection). No element of pressure or coercion should be used to pressurize woman to undergo procedure of sterilization.

STERILIZATION CERTIFICATE

When?

The medical officer of the facility should issue "Certificate of Sterilization" to women 1 month after the surgery or, after the next menstrual period.

Rule out pregnancy before issuing sterilization certificate, if the client does not have her periods even after 1 month of surgery.

For vasectomy, the certificate should be issued after confirming azoospermia in semen analysis done 3 months after surgery.

Discharge slip/card will be considered a valid proof for undergoing slerilization operation for payment of compensation for undergoing sterilization operation.

Format

Sterilization Certificate

Hospital Registration No. (IPD/OPD) ....

1. This is to certify that Smt/Shri .... S/O; W/O Shri. ....
working as .... residing at .... has undergone Minilap Tubectomy—(Interval/Postpartum/Postabortion/Concurrent with other procedures)/ Laparoscopic Tubal Occlusion (Interval/Postabortion/Concurrent with other surgeries)/Vasectomy in this facility/hospital.

(Name of facility/Hospital) on .... by
Dr ....

For Female Sterilization:

2. She has resumed her menstrual cycle (LMP ....) or she has not resumed her menses within the month of sterilization but pregnancy test is negative.

For Male Sterilization:

3. His semen examination undertaken on (Date) .... revealed no sperm (azoospermia).

*Strike out whichever is not applicable.

She/He is therefore certified to be sterile.
Signature of Medical Officer I/c

Name: ....

Date: .... *Seal:*

Note: Client should acknowledge "received" on the duplicate copy before receiving the original copy.

The duplicate to be maintained as a record in the facility as per state norms.

FAILURE OF FEMALE STERILIZATION

Effectiveness of Minilap Tubectomy and Laparoscopic Tubal Occlusion

Minilap tubectomy and laparoscopic tubal occlusion carry a small risk of failure.

- Failure rate with 1 year of sterilization is 0.5%. Over 10 years of use this further goes down to 0.2%. Different techniques have almost same failure rate which is overall low.
- The technique of cutting and tying the cut ends of the fallopian tubes after childbirth (postpartum tubal ligation) is one of the most effective ones.
- The abnormalities of the fallopian tubes; procedural errors and reopening of the tube (recanalization during the healing process may be the cause of failures.
- If occlusion or ligature of tube done only on one side, it may result in failure. In such cases, it should be informed to the client, documented on paper, and signature/thumb impression of the client should be taken on the paper stating that only one tube has been ligated/occluded and sterilization procedure has been unsuccessful.

The sterilization certificate should not be issued, in such cases even if she resumes her menstrual cycle.

Such cases where sterilization certificate has not been issued are *not eligible* for compensation for "failure" under FPIS.

The presence of early and undetected pregnancy at the time of the procedure may be perceived as a failure and must be ruled out carefully.

Tubectomy can be performed, if client still insists, wherein she must be explained that the procedure may not be able to prevent the present pregnancy if existing but can only prevent future pregnancies if any. Surgeon should properly document such cases in case sheet and get it countersigned by the client.

Sterilization certificate can be issued specifying its validity for any subsequent pregnancy and not the current suspected pregnancy.

If the beneficiary is subsequently found to be pregnant on examination then she is *not eligible* for compensation for "failure" under FPIS.

Tubectomy and tubal occlusion do not increase the incidence of ectopic pregnancy. However, if a woman does become pregnant after tubectomy, she is more likely to have an ectopic pregnancy (Pollack 1993).

Any women who have undergone minilap tubectomy and present with symptoms of pregnancy, should be carefully evaluated for ectopic pregnancy.

The failure of sterilization may be due to some technical deficiency in the surgical procedure such as mistaken fallopian tubes with round ligament, not putting Falope rings during laparoscopic tubal occlusion on the full loop of the tubes leading to partial services occlusion, slipping off of the ring after applying or the rings give away (break) after putting on the tubes. Also, there is an element of spontaneous recanalization of the blocked or excised fallopian tube leading to partial or full patency and subsequently leads to pregnancy and failure. The clients are advised to report to the healthcare facility within 2 weeks of missed periods for confirmation about the failure of her sterilization procedure.

She should be offered medical termination of pregnancy and repeat sterilization procedure or be medically supported throughout the pregnancy if she so wishes.

Ectopic pregnancy must be ruled out as female sterilization predisposes to this condition.

FAMILY PLANNING INDEMNITY SCHEME

Family Planning Indemnity Scheme indemnifies all clients of sterilization as also doctors/health facilities conducting sterilization operation in both public and accredited private/NGO sector health facilities for unlikely events of death/complications/failure attributable to sterilization operations. The available benefits under the Family Planning Indemnity Scheme are as under:

- I A Death attributable to sterilization (inclusive of death during process of sterilization operation) in hospital or within 7 days from the date of discharge from the hospital. Rs. 2 lacs
- I B Death attributable to sterilization within 8–30 days from the date of discharge from the hospital. Rs. 50,000/-
- IC Failure of sterilization. Rs 30,000/-
- I D Cost of treatment in hospital and up to 60 days arising out of complication attributable to sterilization operation (inclusive of complication during process of sterilization operation) from the date of discharge. Actual not exceeding Rs. 25,000/-
- II Indemnity per Doctor/Health Facilities but not >4 in a year. Up to Rs. 2 lakh per claim.

Note: The details of the scheme are available in "Manual for Family Planning Indemnity Scheme", available on http://nrhm.gov.in/nrhm-components/rmnch-a/family-planning/schemes.html.

Steps of the Claim Process

District Level Quality Assurance Committee (DQAC) to process the claims arising out of death, complication and failure attributable to sterilization and to be put up to State Level Quality Assurance Committee (SQAC) Beneficiary to file the claims document (within 90 days from the occurrence of event of complications/failures/deaths), stipulated time limit for settlement of claims would be 15 working days in case of death and 21 days in case of others, after submission of all required documents.

CMO/CDMO/CMHO/CDHMO/DMO/Joint Director to duly sign, stamp, and authenticate the claim documents for processing (preferably within 30 days from the date of filing of claims document) SQAC to scrutinize the documents and if required, call for any new and relevant material missing from the recommendation of DQAC. SQAC to review every single case in the state and recommend release of funds to the district, wherever applicable.

REFERENCES

1. Ministry of health and Family Welfare, Government of india. (2006). Standards of female and male sterilization services. [online] Available from https://nhm.gov.in/images/pdf/guidelines/nrhm-guidelines/family-planning/std-for-sterilization-services.pdf [Last accessed December, 2022].
2. Ministry of Health and Family Welfare, Government of India. (2014). Reference manual for female sterilisation. [online] Available from: https://nhm.gov.in/images/pdf/programmes/family-planing/guidelines/Standards_and_Quality_Assurance.pdf [Last accessed December, 2022].

SECTION 3

Guidelines for Use in Selected Population

CHAPTER 14

Postpartum Intrauterine Contraceptive Device

(Col) Bidhan Roy

INTRODUCTION

The time of delivery at a healthcare center offers a unique opportunity to address the need of a practical, affordable, cost-effective, reversible, and universally reproducible by healthcare provider and easily compliable method of contraception. Return of fertility during the postpartum period is unpredictable and hence carries the potential fear of unwanted pregnancies. Postpartum contraception is very unique as it prevents unwanted pregnancies, abortions, and fulfills the need of healthy birth spacing in young couples.[1] Birth spacing optimizes women's health by decreasing maternal mortality and morbidity, preterm birth and low-birthweight babies.

An effective and reversible contraception during the postpartum period has been limited so far. Option for various contraception such as condom, progesterone only pills, lactational amenorrhea method, and tubal ligation may be offered along with the option of postpartum intrauterine device (Copper-T 380 A). Time after delivery is the most motivated time for the decision of contraception but the turmoil of delivery can be a difficult time to decide among the various contraception methods.

Various studies have validated a positive outcome in terms of safety and efficacy with the use of intrauterine contraceptive device after delivery. Postpartum intrauterine contraceptive device (PPIUCD) has been used immediately after delivery of placenta (postplacental) or within 48 hours after delivery and also intraoperatively during cesarean delivery. Hence, counseling should commence during the antenatal period about the various timings of PPIUCD.

Postpartum intrauterine contraceptive device is considered to be a safe and effective contraceptive choice in the postpartum period with manifold benefits.[2] However, acceptability of this method of contraception depends upon substantial counseling by the healthcare provider and counseling should be initiated during the antenatal visits. PPIUCD insertion has the advantage of assurance that the woman is not pregnant, provides a convenient healthcare setting, and is the most motivated time for a clientele for IUCD application. Compared with the interval insertions, postpartum insertions of IUCD neither increase the risk of infection, bleeding, uterine perforations, and subinvolution of uterus.[3,4] Proper insertion techniques and adequate training of the provider have been shown to decrease the expulsion rate in PPIUCD.[5] Ministry of Health and Family Welfare regularly conducts PPIUCD training program in our country. Also, this reversible method of contraception is as effective as that of tubal ligation.[6] Reports of large-scale successful implementation of this family planning method in various countries such as China, Mexico, Egypt, and Kenya have been very encouraging for all of us because of its universal availability and easy implementation in low-resource settings.

Xu J X et al. conducted a study of the PPICUD Copper-T 380 A and they found an expulsion rate of 12.7 per 100 women using ring-forceps insertion. This study showed a discontinuation rate of 1.0 per 100 women users owing to pain and bleeding.[7] It is very important to note that this study found a higher expulsion and discontinuation rate in hand insertion techniques compared to the ring-forceps insertion. No uterine perforation, infection, or pregnancy occurred and hence it was concluded that PPIUCD using Copper-T 380A was suitable for the Chinese women.[7]

In another Chinese study by Xu JX, Connell C, and Chi IC observed the 1-year life-table expulsion rates of PPIUCD inserted at cesarean section are lower than the rates for vaginal insertions after normal delivery.[8] They also concluded that the PPIUCD has the advantage of providing the ideal time as the clients are best motivated after the delivery.[8]

Tatum HJ et al. reported a randomized control study of PPIUCD given within 10 minutes of placental delivery and found an expulsion rate of 13.2 per 100 cases and continuation rate above 80 per 100 users.[9]

Nathalie Kapp and Kathryn M. Curtis concluded a search and systemic review of 15 relevant articles out of 297 related articles on PPIUCD from Medline, Lilacs, and Cochrane Collaboration databases.[10] They compared the outcomes of various postpartum IUD insertion time intervals. They concluded that safety and efficacy of PPIUCD were statistically significant with no postpartum complications. Their search added that some increase in expulsion rates occurred with delayed PPIUCD insertion when compared to immediate PPIUCD insertion.[10] Postplacental placements during cesarean delivery are associated with lower expulsion rates than postplacental vaginal insertions, without increasing rates of postoperative complications.[10]

DISCUSSION

Copper-T 380 A device was developed and marketed first by the Population Council of the United States of America in 1982. They are made up of polyethylene impregnated with barium sulfate. They have 314 mm^3 copper wire on the vertical stem and two 33 mm^2 copper sleeves on each of the two transverse arms. The strings are made up of polyethylene. The approved life span of Cu-T 380 A is 10 years **(Fig. 1)**. Failure rate of Cu-T 380 A is <1 per 100 women users at the end of 1 year of use.

Cu-T 380 A is a low cost and freely available contraceptive in the hospital and requires one-time motivation of the user. With the advent of good road, transport system, and government initiatives, we could see an incremental increase in institutional-based delivery system. Hospital provides an ideal infrastructure and availability of trained personals for the implementation of PPIUCD.

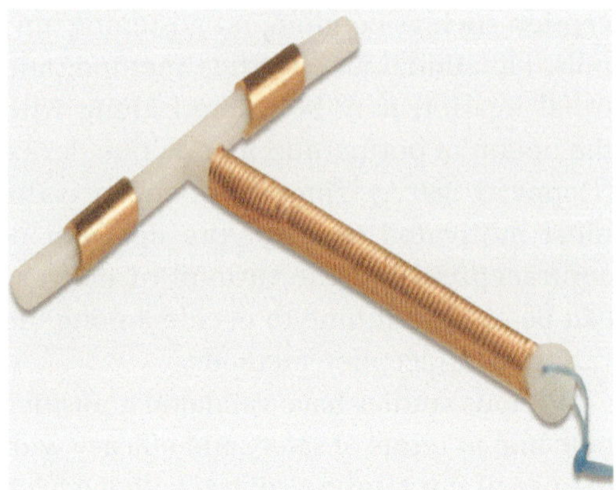

Fig. 1: Cu-T 380 A.

There are many advantages of PPIUCD compared to the other reversible contraceptives in terms of its timing, comfort of the patient, and optimization of already available infrastructure. Discomfort of Cu-T 380 A insertion as PPIUCD is less than during interval period because of the dilated cervix. It does not interfere with the sexual act and has no systemic side effects. The return of fertility is immediately following its removal. Copper-bearing IUDs have no effect on amount or quality of breast milk. It is more effective than other temporary contraceptive methods.

However, certain inherit disadvantages also exist for PPIUCD use, like it needs trained personnel for insertion and subsequent management. Complications such as bleeding, pain, vaginal discharge, infection, perforation, unwanted pregnancy, and ectopic pregnancy can occur. They cannot prevent transmission of HIV like barrier contraceptives (condom). Expulsion of Cu-T 380 A as PPIUCD is higher than during interval period and sometime users are not aware of expulsion leading to failure of contraception.

For our effective fight against population explosion, it is imperative that counseling for various contraceptive measures should be imparted to every lady attending antenatal outpatient department and also to the unbooked cases after in-hospital delivery. In fact, counseling and option of PPIUCD need to be discussed during any opportunistic contact with the patient during the antenatal visit, early labor, and after delivery. A written, informed, and voluntary consent is best to be obtained before the insertion of the postpartum intrauterine contraceptive device keeping in mind the revised WHO eligibility criteria for Cu-T insertion.[6]

Patients with instrumental delivery, prolonged labor, leaking from rupture of membrane for >18 hours, postpartum hemorrhage, uterine anomalies, HIV infection, suspected genital neoplasia, heart disease, and gestational diabetes mellitus are various circumstances wherein PPIUCD is not advised.

Use of long Kelly's placental forceps for insertion ensures high fundal placement of Cu-T **(Fig. 2)**. It is a cheap and easily available instrument. It should be available in every PPIUCD practicing institution. It is to be noted that postdelivery use of uterotonics is not associated with increase in the expulsion rate in PPIUCD. Exclusive breastfeeding should be encouraged as it has the potential of reducing the Cu-T induced bleeding. Patients should be told about the method of detecting expulsions and instructed to return for reinsertion or another method of contraception in the event of expulsion of Cu-T. Long strings of Copper-T if found coming out of vagina should be trimmed off by the patient. Clinical follow-up of the patient should be done at 6 weeks and at 6 months and also as and when required by the patient. Check ultrasonography is a useful method to detect expulsion. Institutional audit of contraceptive failure rate, expulsion rate, and complications such as bleeding

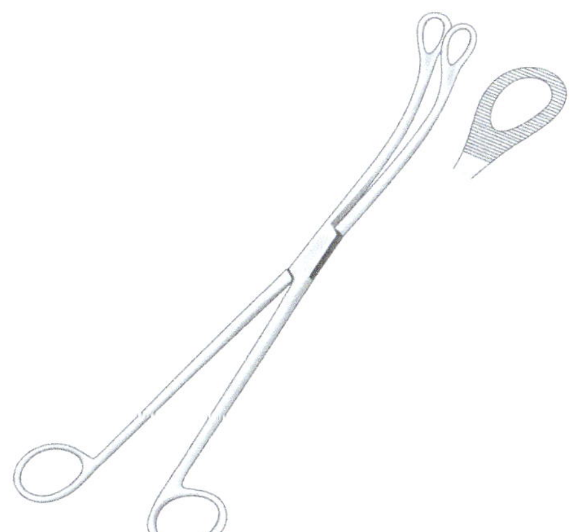

Fig. 2: Kelly's forceps.

per vaginum, infection, perforation, and the acceptance rate among the patient should be kept as a record. A study conducted at our center revealed follow-up patients complaining of bleeding per vaginum in 12% cases, abdominal discomfort in 10% and discharge per vaginum in 5% cases.[11] Mefenamic acid and/or drotaverine tablets are effective for pain abdomen, tranexamic acid tablets for bleeding per vaginum and ofloxacin plus ornidazole along with clotrimazole/clindamycin vaginal pessary for vaginal discharge are recommended for respective complaints during the follow-up period. Reassurance about these temporary initial signs and symptoms should be an important part of the counseling. All such minor ailments are generally managed conservatively without any untoward complications. Our study figured a removal rate of 13% including the expulsion rate of 4% and 87% continuation rate[11] compared to 82% as reported in other studies.[12-14] A standard follow-up management of complaints should be available in the hospital and follow-up is an important component for the success of the PPIUCD program.[15]

CONCLUSION

Hospitals are ideal settings for this low cost, easily available, safe, effective, and reversible contraceptive method. Health awareness about PPIUCD in the hospital by infographics increases the acceptance rate among the clientele. Thus, PPIUCD offers a unique opportunity for all the hospital delivery patients and is a major policy shift in the concept of contraception and population control within the available resources. Thus, there is more benefit to the reproductive population without any increase in the cost or extra burden to our existing infrastructure.

However, counseling and training of the care provider (doctors, nurses, and health staffs) of a hospital form integral part in the success of this noble program. Awareness about this postpartum contraceptive program through mass media will help in convincing and establishing the core benefits to population at large. Proactive advocacy of postpartum contraception has many fold health benefits and averts complications of unwanted pregnancies.

REFERENCES

1. The Global Health Observatory. Unmet need for family planning. Geneva: World Health Organization.
2. Grimes DA, Lopez LM, Schulz KF, Van Vliet HAAM, Stanwood NL. Immediate post-partum insertion of intrauterine devices. Cochrane Database Syst Rev. 2010;5: CD003036.
3. Marai W. Lower genital tract infections among pregnant women: a review. East Africa Med J. 2001;78(11):581-5.
4. Kurewa NE, Mapingure MP, Munjoma MW, Chirenje MZ, Rusakaniko S, Stray-Pedersen B. The burden and risk factors of sexually transmitted infections and reproductive tract infections among pregnant women in Zimbabwe. BioMed Central Infect Dis. 2010;10:127.
5. Thiery M, Van Kets H, Van Der Pas H. Immediate post placental IUD insertion: the expulsion problems. Contraception. 1985; 31;331-49.
6. Bluestone J, Chase R, Lu ER. (2006). IUCD Guidelines for family planning: a problem-solving reference manual, 3rd edition. [online] Available from https://www.semanticscholar.org/paper/IUD-guidelines-for-family-planning-service-a-3rd-Bluestone-Chase/5e24233cb75affb00c4073d7241b2dd7b271398c [Last accessed November, 2022].
7. Xu JX, Rivera R, Dunson TR, Zhuang LQ, Yang XL, Ma GT, et al. A comparative study

of two techniques used in immediate post placental insertion of Copper-T380A in Shanghai, People's Republic of China. Adv Contracept. 1994;10(1):71-82.

8. Xu JX, Connell C, Chi IC. Immediate postpartum intrauterine device insertion—a report on the Chinese experience. Adv Contracept.19928(4):281-90.
9. Tatum HJ, Beltran RS, Ramos R, Van Kets H, Sivin I, Schmidt FH. Immediate post placental insertion of Gyne-T 380 postpartum intrauterine contraceptive devices: randomized study. Am J Obstet Gynecol. 1996;175(5): 1231-5.
10. Kapp N, Curtis KM. Intrauterine device insertion during the postpartum period: a systemic review. Contraception. 2009;80(4): 327-36.
11. Bidhan R, Shivakumar RN, Paprikar MM. Study the safety and efficacy of post-partum intrauterine contraceptive device. Int J Res Rev. 2019;6(10):252-8.
12. Chen BA, Hayes JL, Hohmann HL, Perriera LK, Reeves MF, Creinin MD. A randomized trial of post placental compared to delayed insertion of the levonorgestrel-releasing intrauterine device after vaginal delivery. Contraception. 2009;80(2):205.
13. Peipert JF, Zhao Q, Allsworth JE, Petrosky E, Madden T, Eisenberg D. Continuation and satisfaction of reversible contraception. Obstet Gynecol. 2011;117(5):1105-13.
14. Celen S, Moroy P, Sucak A, Aktulay A, Danisman N. Clinical outcomes of early post placental insertion of intrauterine contraceptive devices. Contraception. 2004;69:279-82.
15. World Health Organization. (2013). Programming strategies for post-partum family planning: Maternal and Child health Integrated program: 2013: Reference manual by WHO and USAID. [online] Available from: https://apps.who.int/iris/bitstream/handle/10665/93680/9789241506496_eng.pdf [Last accessed November, 2022].

CHAPTER 15

Contraceptives for Transgender Individuals

(Col) Bidhan Roy

INTRODUCTION

Transgenderism involves a complex spectrum of biological, cultural, and environmental influences upon an individual. Transgender individuals have a gender identity or gender expression that differs from the sex that they are assigned at birth. Transgender females (TGF) are those who live or identify as females but are being labeled as male at birth. Transgender males (TGM) are those who live or identify as males but are being labeled as female at birth.

As per 2011 census, there are around 488,000 transgender (third gender) population in India. While in the United States, there were 1,040,000 transgender population in 2016. Worldwide, there are a lot of myths and misconceptions about healthcare perceptions for transgender individuals. Presence of trans-friendly healthcare infrastructure and trained healthcare providers should be included in healthcare programs of all nations. Thus, there is a felt need of universal strategic planning that addresses medical aid, societal acceptance and legal framework for transgender individuals. Gynecological care toward transgender individuals is an integral part of their healthcare management. It is desired that healthcare providers bring awareness and get trained themselves toward the special contraceptive attention that is required for the transgender individuals for healthy sexual practice. This article attempts to put forward an update on contraceptive care for transgender individuals.

DEFINITION

- Gender expression is the external appearance of a person such as body habitus, clothing, behavior, etc., whereas a person's intrinsic feeling of being male, female, or an alternate gender is designated as the gender identity.
- Gender identity of an individual is determined by the interplay of genetic, gonadal, and phenotypic sex along with environmental influences.
- Sexual orientation implies an inherent physical or emotional component of sexual behavior and it should not be labeled as per the gender identity or gender expression.

GYNECOLOGICAL CARE

Appropriate and timely initiation of hormonal therapy for transgender individuals plays a very important role in their mental, physical, and social wellbeing. An adolescent transgender requires hormone suppression and then hormone induction therapy after attainment of Tanner stage 2. Clinical assessment for underlying gender dysphoria, venous thromboembolism risk, hepatic disorders, and cardiovascular issues should be done followed by biochemical and baseline hormonal investigations. Hormonal suppression during pubertal stage is done by gonadotropin-releasing hormone (GnRH) analog (leuprolide) along with calcium and vitamin D supplements. Thereafter, puberty induction in TG females is done by the use of estrogen while puberty induction for TG males is done by use of testosterone. Evolving gender-assigning-surgeries have opened a new frontier of surgical dimension in aid of transgender population.

Contraceptive need arises when a transgender individual develops sexual relationship with a cisgender individual. The hormonal suppression or reaffirming therapy does decrease the fertility potential but does not translate into absolute contraception and may generate a teratogenic environment (e.g., use of testosterone). Eligibility criteria for contraceptives in transgender individuals represent a special subset wherein more research is needed. Survey among transgender individuals reveal lack of awareness about the need of contraception. Myths and misconception about fertility and pregnancy risk exist in the transgender community and require deep understanding and new deliberations in our existing practice of medicine. Correct alignment of the nature of contraceptive in them is essential to avoid dysphoria, unwanted pregnancy, and neurocognitive development. Side effects of various contraceptives should be disclosed before giving them to the transgender clientele so as to increase the acceptance and compliance.

TRANSGENDER FEMALE

Healthy sexual practices form an integral aspect of multidisciplinary healthcare management. The objective of gender affirming hormone therapy for TG female is to develop the female secondary sexual characteristics such as breast development, female pattern of subcutaneous fat distribution, and to suppress male secondary sexual characteristics like decrease in muscle mass, decrease in testicular volume, and decrease in facial and bodily hair growth.

Gender affirming hormone therapy is not a reliable form of contraception and any antiandrogen drug is teratogenic. A TG female having sexual relationships with a cisgender female should use barrier contraceptive measures and alternatively the cisgender partner may use any form of contraceptives. Estrogen use in TG females increases the risk of venous thromboembolism, hypertriglyceridemia, hyperprolactinemia, hyperglycemia, low bone mass, gallstones, weight gain, cardiovascular disease, and decreased libido. Oral preparation of estrogen has got the higher complication rate than the transdermal patch. Hence, modifiable risk factors such as obesity, hypertension, smoking, and sedentary habits should be corrected while on hormonal treatment. Communication and counseling are the pillars of successful outcome of contraceptive care in transgender individuals.

TRANSGENDER MALE

Transgender males need to be on gender reaffirming hormonal therapy after completion of puberty so as to develop male secondary sexual characteristics. TG males who are on gender affirming hormonal therapy and in a sexual relationship with a cisgender male should use nonhormonal intrauterine devices or a barrier contraceptive. In such circumstances, contraceptive measures should continue till gender assigning-surgeries like hysterectomy and bilateral salpingo-ophorectomy are done.

If pregnancy is not desired, then TG males who are not on gender reaffirming hormonal therapy and are in sexual relationship with a cisgender male should use some contraceptives such as combined hormonal pills, hormonal or nonhormonal intrauterine devices, contraceptive patches, vaginal contraceptive rings, and long-acting reversible contraceptive implants (LARC). Side effects of each one of them are variable and prolonged amenorrhea is a desirable side-effect in this subset of third gender. Contraceptive cover should continue till hysterectomy and bilateral salpingo-ophorectomy are accomplished.

CONCLUSION

Goal of contraceptive care is to integrate healthy transgenders into general community. With widening legal and societal acceptance, there has been a justified demand of safe and better healthcare access to transgender individuals. It is time to understand and address health issues of transgender people in of our society.

FURTHER READING

1. Chapkin SR, Kim F. Ten most important things to know about caring for transgender patients. Am J Med. 2017;130(11):1238-45.
2. Deutsch MB, Bhakri V, Kubicek K. Effects of cross-sex hormone treatment on transgender women and men. Obstet Gynecol. 2015; 125(3):605-10.
3. Gorin-Lazard A, Baumstarck K, Boyer L, Maquigneau A, Penochet JC, Pringuey D, et al. Hormonal therapy is associated with better self-esteem, mood and quality of life in transsexuals. J Nerv Ment Dis. 2013;201(11):996-1000.
4. Hembree WC, Cohen-Kettenis PT, Gooren L, Hannema SE, Meyer WJ, Murad MH, et al. Endocrine treatment of gender-dysphoric/gender-incongruent persons: an Endocrine Society Clinical Practice guideline. J Clin Endocrinol Metab. 2017;102(11):3869-903.
5. Irwg M. Clinical dilemmas in the management of transgender men. Curr Opin. 2017; 24(3):233-9.
6. Irwig M. Testosterone therapy for transgender men. Lancet Diabetes Endocrinol. 2017;5(4): 301-11.
7. Lee PA, Houk CP, Ahmed SF, Hughes IA. Consensus statement on management of intersex disorders. International Consensus Conference on Intersex. Paediatrics. 2006; 118:e488.
8. Unger CA. Care of the transgender patient: the role of the gynecologist. Obstet Gynecol. 2014;210(1):16-26.
9. Weinand JD, Safer JD. Hormone therapy in transgender adults is safe with provider supervision: a review of hormone therapy sequelae for transgender individuals. J Clin Transl Endocrinol. 2015;2(2):55-60.
10. Weyers S, De Sutter P, Hoebeke S, Monstrey G, T Sjoen G, Verstraelen H, et al. Gynecological aspects of the treatment and follow-up of transsexual men and women. Facts Views Vis Obgyn. 2010;2(1):35-54.
11. World Professional Association for Transgender Health. (2018). Standards of care for the health of transsexual, transgender and gender nonconforming people. [online] Available from http://www.wpath.org/site [Last accessed November, 2022].

CHAPTER

16 Safety Issues of Contraceptives for Women over 35 Years

Indrani Mukhopadhyay, Uma Wankhede

INTRODUCTION

There are many birth control options available currently, but these require individualization as per the women depending on her desire for future fertility and her age. With more and more women achieving financial independence, there is an ever-changing role being played by today's women in society. This is not only empowering the women socially but also putting a greater professional responsibility, leading to a conscious decision to delay fertility and conception beyond 30 years of age. Hence, birth control methods for elderly women beyond 35 years of age and those with medical conditions have become an increasingly important topic of concern. It becomes important to discuss the suitability and safety of each of these contraceptive methods. Also, contraceptive use is a greater concern in perimenopausal women with irregular ovulatory cycles and resultant unintended pregnancies. Since decades, it was the oral contraception that was routinely prescribed, but lately, there are diverse options available for women. Because of the concerns regarding increased risk of venous thromboembolism (VTE), cardiovascular complications, and poor compliance, the long-acting progesterone-only contraceptives with one-time use are going to be the way forward in contraception.

DISCUSSION

According to international guidelines, age is not an independent contraindicating factor for contraceptive methods. The nonhormonal and progestin-only methods are safe for women with any medical contraindication for estrogens. For women who are using hormonal contraceptives, onset of menopause can be assumed at age 55.[1] The fecundity has been variably reported from 0.2 for women less than 35 years of age, compared with 0.12 for women 35–40 years and 0.06 for women over 40 years.[2] All unintended pregnancies in ladies beyond 35 years involve higher obstetrical risks and their prevalence among women aged 35 years or more is up to 31.3%.[3] Hence in this scenario, with larger health risks involved, it is imperative to weigh the risks and benefits before beginning with any form of contraception **(Table 1)**.

UNITED KINGDOM ELIGIBILITY CRITERIA FOR USE OF CONTRACEPTION AMONG ELDERLY WOMEN

The United Kingdom (UK) eligibility criteria for use of contraception among elderly women with respect to individual method of contraception **(Table 2)**.

TABLE 1: Special considerations about method of choice in elderly women above 35 years as per the WHO.[4]

<table>
<tr>
<td>Combined hormonal methods that include COCs, monthly injectables, combined patch, and combined vaginal ring
• Women >35 years who smoke, regardless of how much, should not use COCs, the patch, or the combined vaginal ring
• Women aged 35 years and older who smoke 15 or more cigarettes a day should not use monthly injectables
• Women aged 35 years or older should not use COCs, monthly injectables, the patch, or the combined vaginal ring if they have migraine headaches (whether with migraine aura or not)</td>
<td>Progestin-only methods that include progestin-only pills, progestin-only injectables, and implants
• For women who cannot use methods with estrogen
• During use, DMPA decreases bone mineral density, slightly increasing the risk of developing osteoporosis and bone fractures, after menopause. WHO has concluded that this decrease in bone mineral density does not place age or time limits on use of DMPA</td>
<td>Emergency contraceptive pills can be used by women of any age, including those who cannot use hormonal methods on a continuing basis</td>
<td>Female sterilization and vasectomy
• May be a good choice for older women and their partners who know they will not want more children
• Some women may have conditions that may cause delay or require caution for female sterilization</td>
</tr>
<tr>
<td>Intrauterine device that includes copper-bearing IUDs and LNG-IUDs:
• Expulsion rates fall as women grow older and are lowest in women over 40 years of age
• Insertion may be more difficult due to tightening of the cervical canal</td>
<td>Fertility awareness methods:
• Lack of regular cycles before menopause makes it more difficult to use these methods reliably</td>
<td colspan="2">Male and female condoms, diaphragms, spermicides, cervical caps, and withdrawal:
• Protect older women well because of women's reduced fertility in the years before menopause
• Affordable and convenient for women who may not have sex often</td>
</tr>
</table>

(COC: combined oral contraceptive; DMPA: depot medroxyprogesterone acetate; WHO: World Health organization)

Levonorgestrel-releasing Intrauterine System (Mirena®)

Levonorgestrel-releasing intrauterine system (LNG-IUS) is the progesterone-only intrauterine device (IUD) that helps in a regular release of progesterone—levonorgestrel (LNG). LNG-IUS may confer a protective effect against ovarian and endometrial cancer. Current guidance contraindicates use of a LNG-IUS for women with previous or current breast cancer. Evidence suggests that there is little or no increased risk of VTE or myocardial infarction (MI) associated with the use of a LNG-IUS.[6]

TABLE 2: The UK eligibility criteria for contraceptive use in women above 35 years or with a medical condition.[5]

Condition	Category					
	Cu IUD	Levonorgestrel-releasing IUD	Implant	DMPA	POP	CHC
Postpartum (breastfeeding):						
• 21 to <30 days postpartum With other risk factors for VTE (e.g., age ≥35 years, previous VTE, thrombophilia, immobility, transfusion at delivery, peripartum cardiomyopathy, BMI ≥30 kg/m², postpartum hemorrhage, postcesarean delivery, preeclampsia, or smoking)	–	–	Benefits outweigh risks	Benefits outweigh risks	Benefits outweigh risks	Unacceptable risk
• 30–42 days postpartum With other risk factors for VTE (e.g., age ≥35 years, previous VTE, thrombophilia, immobility, transfusion at delivery, peripartum cardiomyopathy, BMI ≥30 kg/m², postpartum hemorrhage, postcesarean delivery, preeclampsia, or smoking)	–	–	No restriction	No restriction	No restriction	Unacceptable risk
Postpartum (nonbreastfeeding women)						
• 21–42 days postpartum With other risk factors for VTE (e.g., age ≥35 years, previous VTE, thrombophilia, immobility, transfusion at delivery, peripartum cardiomyopathy, BMI ≥30 kg/m², postpartum hemorrhage, postcesarean delivery, preeclampsia, or smoking)	–	–	No restriction	No restriction	No restriction	Unacceptable risk

Contd...

Contd...

Condition	Category					
	Cu IUD	**Levonorgestrel-releasing IUD**	**Implant**	**DMPA**	**POP**	**CHC**
Smoking (age > 35 years)						
• <15 cigarettes per day	• No restriction	• No restriction	• No restriction	• No restriction	• No restriction	• Risks outweigh benefits
• >15 cigarettes per day	• No restriction	• Unacceptable risk	• Unacceptable risk	• Unacceptable risk	• Unacceptable risk	• Unacceptable risk
Multiple risk factors for atherosclerotic cardiovascular disease (e.g., older age, smoking, diabetes, hypertension, low HDL, high LDL, or high triglyceride levels)	No restriction	Benefits outweigh risks	Benefits outweigh risks	Risks outweigh benefits	Benefits outweigh risks	Risks outweigh benefits/ unacceptable risk
Obesity (BMI ≥30 kg/m²)	No restriction	No restriction	No restriction	No restriction	No restriction	Benefits outweigh risks
Hypertension:						
• Adequately controlled hypertension	• No restriction	• No restriction	• No restriction	• Benefits outweigh risks	• No restriction	• Risks outweigh benefits
• Elevated blood pressure levels (properly taken measurements)	• No restriction	• No restriction	• No restriction	• Benefits outweigh risks	• No restriction	• Risks outweigh benefits
– Systolic 140–159 mm Hg or diastolic 90–99 mm Hg	• No restriction	• Benefits outweigh risks	• Benefits outweigh risks	• Risks outweigh benefits	• No restriction	• Unacceptable risk
– Systolic ≥ 160 mm Hg or diastolic ≥ 100 mm Hg	• No restriction	• Benefits outweigh risks	• Benefits outweigh risks	• Risks outweigh benefits	• Benefits outweigh risks	• Unacceptable risk
• Vascular disease						
Diabetes:						
• Nonvascular disease	• No restriction	• Benefits outweigh risks	• Benefits outweigh risks	• Benefits outweigh risks	• Benefits outweigh risks	• Benefits outweigh risks
• With vascular disease	• No restriction	• Benefits outweigh risks	• Benefits outweigh risks	• Risks outweigh benefits	• Benefits outweigh risks	• Unacceptable risk

Contd...

Contd...

Condition	***Category***					
	Cu IUD	***Levonorgestrel-releasing IUD***	***Implant***	***DMPA***	***POP***	***CHC***
Stroke	No restriction	Benefits outweigh risks	Benefits outweigh risks	Risks outweigh benefits	Benefits outweigh risks	Unacceptable risk
Current/past ischemic heart disease	No restriction	Benefits outweigh risks	Benefits outweigh risks	Risks outweigh benefits	Benefits outweigh risks	Unacceptable risk
Unexplained vaginal bleeding (suspicious for serious condition) before evaluation	Unacceptable risk	Unacceptable risk	Risks outweigh benefits	Risks outweigh benefits	Benefits outweigh risks	Benefits outweigh risks
Endometrial hyperplasia	No restriction	No restriction	No restriction	No restriction	No restriction	No restriction
Endometrial cancer	Unacceptable risk	Unacceptable risk	No restriction	No restriction	No restriction	No restriction
Ovarian cancer	No restriction	No restriction	No restriction	No restriction	No restriction	No restriction
Endometriosis	Benefits outweigh risks	No restriction	No restriction	No restriction	No restriction	No restriction
Benign ovarian tumors (including cysts)	No restriction	No restriction	No restriction	No restriction	No restriction	No restriction

(BMI: body mass index; CHC: combined hormonal contraceptive; Cu IUD: copper intrauterine device; DMPA: depot medroxyprogesterone acetate; HDL: high-density lipoprotein; LDL: low-density lipoprotein; POP: progestogen-only pill; US: United States; VTE: venous thromboembolism)

The Faculty of Sexual and Reproductive Healthcare (FSRH) supports the extended use of a Mirena® 52 mg LNG-IUS for contraception until the age of 55 years if inserted at age 45 years or over, provided it is not being used as the progestogen replacement therapy [component of hormone replacement therapy (HRT)] for endometrial protection.

Nexplanon

Nexplanon is a progesterone-only implant (IMP) that lasts for 3 years. This is the most effective form of contraception available with a 0.05% failure rate[7] and there is no age restriction to its use. There are episodes of spotting/no periods with this form of contraception. The progestogen-only IMP is not associated with increased risks of VTE, stroke, or MI and has not been shown to affect bone mineral density (BMD). The available evidence suggests no significant increase in risk of breast cancer. Evidence is too limited to inform whether there is any association between use of the etonogestrel IMP (ENG-IMP) and risk of ovarian, endometrial, or cervical cancer.[8]

Depot Medroxyprogesterone

Currently, two depot medroxyprogesterone acetate (DMPA) contraceptive injections are in common use in the DepoProvera®/DMPA/Antara and Sayana Press. It may cause irregular cycles, irregular ovulation, and irregular bleeding episodes. Studies indicate that DMPA may have a potentially protective effect on risk of endometrial or ovarian cancer. Women using DMPA experience initial bone loss due to the hypoestrogenic effects of DMPA. There is limited evidence regarding stroke and MI risk for women using DMPA. There is possibly a weak association between current use and breast cancer. Women of all ages using DMPA should be reviewed every 2 years to assess the benefits and risks of use.[9] Women over 50 years should be counseled on alternative methods of contraception.

COMBINED HORMONAL CONTRACEPTIVE[10]

Combined hormonal contraceptives (CHCs) include combined oral pills, patches, and rings. At the age of 50 years, they should be advised to switch from CHC to a noninjectable progestogen-only contraception (POC) or a nonhormonal method as the risks of CHC generally outweigh the contraceptive benefits. Women who smoke should be advised to stop CHC at age the age of 35 years as this is the age at which excess risk of mortality becomes significant. Once a woman over 35 years has stopped smoking for >1 year, then use of CHC becomes less restrictive. Combined oral contraceptive (COC) with ≤30 µg ethinylestradiol should be considered first-line COC preparations for women over 40 due to the potentially lower risks of VTE, cardiovascular disease, and stroke. COC is associated with a reduced risk of ovarian and endometrial cancer that lasts for several decades after cessation. Studies have found a slight increased risk of breast cancer among women using COC but with no significant risk of breast cancer by 10 years after cessation.

PROGESTERONE-ONLY PILLS

Formulations either include desogestrel (DSG), norethisterone, or LNG. Women using a DSG pill are more likely to become anovulatory. Women can be informed that the progestogen-only pill (POP) is not associated with increased risks of VTE, stroke, or MI and has not been shown to affect BMD. One consideration—over 40 years is the potential for altered bleeding patterns.[11] The available evidence does not support an association between breast cancer and POP use.[12]

BARRIER CONTRACEPTIVES

Barrier methods include male condoms, female condoms, diaphragms, and cervical caps. There are no age restrictions to the use of barrier methods and there are few contraindications.[13] Barrier methods often have high effectiveness in women over 40 years due to declining fertility and more consistent usage.

What is to be remembered that none of them prevent from sexually transmitted diseases.

CONCLUSION

The contraceptives as per the World Health organization (WHO), categorized as the "top-tier" methods with respect to effectiveness are the copper IUDs, progestin IUDs, progestin IMPs, and sterilization.[3] They are preferred only after weighing the risk and benefit concerns. These methods are associated with failure rates of less than 1% with typical use in the first year of use. However because of decreasing fertility, contraceptive failure rates are lower among the elderly women and hence less effective; short-acting methods such as oral contraceptives or coitally dependent methods (male and female condoms, diaphragms, and emergency contraception) may also be acceptable. It is the responsibility of the provider to tailor contraceptive options to the woman's needs and to guide her in selecting the best method for the lady rather than prescribing a single method. Furthermore, providers need to follow the medical philosophy, "first, do no harm" on some occasions when a woman's medical condition was too "high risk" for contraception, and hence should avoid any form of contraception in such situations. Voluntary informed choice of contraceptive methods is an essential guiding principle to the successful use of contraceptive methods.

REFERENCES

1. Allen RH, Cwiak CA, Kaunitz AM. Contraception in women over 40 years of age. CMAJ. 2013;185(7):565-73.
2. Kang BM, Wu TC. Effect of age on intrauterine insemination with frozen donor sperm. Obstet Gynecol. 1996;88:93-8.
3. Dutta M, Shekhar C, Prashad L. Level, Trend and Correlates of Mistimed and Unwanted Pregnancies among Currently Pregnant Ever Married Women in India. PLoS One. 2015;10(12):e0144400.
4. Johns Hopkins Bloomberg School of Public Health/Center for Communication Programs, World Health Organization. (2018). Family Planning: A Global Handbook for Providers, 3rd edition. [online] Available from: https://fphandbook.org/sites/default/files/global-handbook-2018-full-web.pdf [Last accessed January, 2024].
5. Curtis KM, Tepper NK, Jatlaoui TC, Berry-Bibee E, Horton LG, Zapata LB, et al. (2016). U.S. Medical Eligibility Criteria for Contraceptive Use. [online] Available from: https://www.cdc.gov/mmwr/volumes/65/rr/rr6503a1.htm [Last accessed January, 2024].
6. FSRH. (2023). FSRH Guideline Intrauterine Contraception. [online] Available from: https://www.fsrh.org/documents/ceuguidanceintrauterinecontraception/fsrh-clinical-guideline-intrauterine-contraception-mar23-amended-11jul2023-.pdf [Last accessed January, 2024].
7. Hou MY, McNicholas C, Creinin MD. Combined oral contraceptive treatment for bleeding complaints with the etonogestrel contraceptive implant: a randomised controlled trial. Eur J Contracept Reprod Health Care. 2016;21:361-6.
8. FSRH. (2021). FSRH Clinical Guideline: Progestogen-only Implants. [online] Available from: https://www.fsrh.org/documents/cec-ceu-guidance-implants-feb-2014/ [Last accessed January, 2024].
9. FSRH. (2014). FSRH Clinical Guideline: Progestogen-only Injectable Contraception. [online] Available from: https://www.

fsrh.org/documents/cec-ceu-guidance-injectables-dec-2014/ [Last accessed January, 2024].

10. FSRH. (2017). FSRH Guideline Contraception for Women Aged Over 40 Years. [online] Available from: https://www.fsrh.org/documents/fsrh-guidance-contraception-for-women-aged-over-40-years-2017/ [Last accessed January, 2024].
11. Faculty of Sexual & Reproductive Healthcare (FSRH). (2015). Progestogen-only Pills. Available from: https://www.fsrh.org/standards-and-guidance/fsrh-guidelines-and-statements/method-specific/progestogen-only-pills/ [Last accessed January, 2024].
12. Samson M, Porter N, Orekoya O, Hebert JR, Adams SA, Bennett CL, et al. Progestin and breast cancer risk: a systematic review. Breast Cancer Res Treat. 2016;155:3-12.
13. Faculty of Sexual & Reproductive Healthcare (FSRH). (2012). FSRH Clinical Guideline: Barrier Methods for Contraception and STI Prevention. [online] Available from: https://www.fsrh.org/standards-and-guidance/documents/ceuguidancebarriermethod-scontraceptionsdi/ [Last accessed January, 2024].

CHAPTER 17

Perimenopausal Women

Uma Wankhede, Swati Gurav

INTRODUCTION

Contraception is the integral part of women's healthcare. Preventing unwanted pregnancies is crucial for women at all ages, particularly perimenopausal women to avoid pregnancy with complications, such as miscarriage high blood pressure diabetes and to reduce the chance of unsafe abortions. The risk of ectopic pregnancies also rises with age. During the perimenopause period, fertility declines however if contraception is not used it increases unintended pregnancies. Hence women should continue contraception till menopause. Menopause is defined as the absence of menses for 2 years in women below age 50 and for 1 year in women over age of 50 years.[1] During perimenopause women might have symptoms, such as hot flashes, night sweats, joint and muscle pain, vaginal dryness, and mood changes. Due to a fall in estrogen levels during perimenopause women may have menstrual irregularities.

DIAGNOSIS OF PERIMENOPAUSE

Over 45 years of age, the diagnosis of perimenopause can be made without laboratory tests in women who have vasomotor symptoms and irregular periods. The serum follicle-stimulating hormone (FSH) test is used to diagnose menopause in women 40–45 years with menopausal symptoms including changes in their menstrual cycle and in women under 40 years of age in whom menopause is suspected. Combine oral contraceptives should be stopped 2 weeks prior to testing due to their effect on FSH level.

Contraception does not affect the timing and duration of menopause but may mask symptoms of perimenopause or menopause. Hormone replacement therapy (HRT) should be used along with contraceptives to avoid unwanted pregnancy. Prerequisites: Before starting any contraception detailed personal family and sexual history should be taken and pregnancy must be ruled out. Body mass index should be calculated and blood pressure to be checked before the start of any contraception. Sexually transmitted diseases (STI) screening should be offered to all women especially prior to the insertion of an intrauterine device (IUD). Pelvic examination is one of the prerequisites before inserting an IUD. Cervical cytology should be offered. All methods of contraception are available to perimenopausal women including natural methods, withdrawal, male, female condoms, combined hormonal contraceptives (pill, patch, and ring), contraceptive injections, contraceptive implants, progestogen-only methods [progestin-only pills (POP) or mini pill], intrauterine system, and other contraceptive methods, such as IUD, male and female sterilization, and emergency contraception.

PAST, PRESENT, AND FUTURE ABOUT PERIMENOPAUSAL CONTRACEPTION

Past

Because of the decline in natural fertility after the mid-30s, and irregular periods with reduced libido many women wrongly assumed contraception could be stopped.

Present

Contraception must be used alongside HRT to avoid unplanned pregnancy. Combined progestogen and estrogen HRT must be used in women with an intact uterus. Contraception must be used alongside HRT to avoid unplanned conception. There is limited data about progestogen in most hormonal contraception methods that provide endometrial protection. Along with contraception, Mirena levonorgestrel (LNG)-releasing intrauterine system (IUS) (52 mg IUS) also provides endometrial protection as part of an HRT regimen.

Future

Future studies are required regarding the safety of combined oral contraceptives (COCs) containing natural estrogens in comparison with traditional oral contraceptives. The association of depot medroxyprogesterone acetate (DMPA) in women over 40 years of age and the risk of osteoporotic fractures need to be studied. Future research regarding intrauterine contraception, microchip drug release technology, progesterone receptor modulators, male contraception, and vaccines is needed.

Barrier methods barrier methods include male condoms, female condoms, diaphragms, and cervical caps.

Male Condoms

Male condoms[2] are widely available and the majority is made up of latex rubber. The use of the male condom is limited if male partner suffers from erectile problems.

THE FEMALE CONDOM (FEMIDOM)

These are less widely available. The higher cost is one of the causes for its limited use. The vaginal dryness can be treated by the use of water-based lubricant at the time of sex.

- *The diaphragm and cervical cap:* Silicon diaphragm can be one of the appropriate methods but it does not prevent STI.
- *Combined hormonal methods (CHC):* There are three types of combined hormonal contraceptives which include (1) combined oral contraceptive pill (COC pill, combined transdermal patch—Evra, and combined vaginal ring—Nuvaring). CHC regimens usually comprise 21 days of active hormones followed by a hormone-free interval of 7 days. Vaginal ring is 4 mm thick and 54 mm in diameter. The vaginal rings release, on average, 120 µg/day of etonogestrel and 15 µg/day of ethinylestradiol (EE) over a 3-week period of use.[3]
- Estrogen-containing pills can be given to women until 50 years if there are no health risks (e.g., smoking, obesity, and high blood pressure) which could lead to heart stroke or blood clotting problems. Combined hormonal methods is generally stopped to women who smoke, have hypertension, or have body mass index (BMI) >35 years.[1] Due to reduced effect on laboratory coagulation tests pills containing estradiol or estradiol valerate can be used in place of EE. The additional benefit from continuous use of combined

pills for 3 months by skipping hormone-free breaks is to reduce blood loss for women with heavy menstrual bleeding. Combined hormonal method use offers additional benefits beyond contraception such as (1) regularization of menstrual bleeding, reduction in dysmenorrhea and pelvic pain; (2) relief of menopausal symptoms such as hot flushes and night sweats; and (3) prevention of bone loss due to demineralization and increasing bone mineral density. Combined hormonal method users have a reduced risk of endometrial, ovarian, and colorectal cancers. Generally, CHC is appropriate contraception for healthy perimenopausal women.

Risks

Women using CHC with the lowest hormonal dose (20 μg EE and LNG 35 μg) have a reduced risk of venous thromboembolism, stroke, and myocardial infarction (MI).

Combined Oral Contraception

Most COC is a combination that contains both synthetic estrogen and progestin. Low-dose COC usually contains between 20 and 35 μg of synthetic estrogen (EE) in combination with synthetic newer-generation progestin. The majority of COC products are monophasic; that is, all pills in the packet contain the same dose of estrogen and progestogen. Multiphasic (variable dose) COC is also available in which the dose of either or both steroid hormones varies during the pill cycle.

Prerequisite

A thorough history and physical examination should be done prior to the start of COC to rule out contraindications (e.g., migraine, DVT, etc.). Body mass index, breast examination, and blood pressure should be checked. For simplicity, 21 hormone pills are taken starting from day one of menses followed by pill free break of 7 days.

Mechanism of Action

Inhibition of ovulation and alteration of cervical mucus.[3]

The extended regimen can be useful for heavy menstrual bleeding that occurs in the late 40s where COCs are continuously given for 84 days of estrogen and progestin followed by 7 days of placebo.[3] This has shown to have advantages such as decreased incidence of pelvic pain, headaches, bloating/swelling, breast tenderness, improvement in symptoms of endometriosis, and polycystic ovary syndrome. Combined oral contraceptives can also reduce vasomotor symptoms and can be considered especially important for perimenopausal women with vasomotor symptoms. Combined oral contraceptives are also useful for bone protection if they are taken by women in their 40s. Combined oral contraceptives can be offered to women up to the age of 50 years and have no risk for cardiovascular disease, such as family history, past deep venous thrombosis, hypertension, diabetes, dyslipidemia, and varicose vein.[1]

Special Consideration

Combined oral contraceptive containing LNG is associated with a lower risk of venous thromboembolism (VTE) than using COC with other progestin.

Noncontraceptive Benefits

Combined oral contraceptives are associated with a reduced risk of ovarian and endometrial cancer that lasts for several decades after cessation. Perimenopausal women also have benefits of COCs which are common to all ages such as reducing dysmenorrhea, anemia, pelvic infection, relief of symptoms of premenstrual syndrome, endometriosis, uterine fibroid, and functional ovarian cyst.

Side Effects

Unexpected breakthrough bleeding can be due to reduced absorption during vomiting, diarrhea, or simultaneous intake of enzyme inducers. Excessive weight gain, mood changes, severe headache, mastalgia, and rise in blood pressure.

Contraindication

Absolute contraindication: Past history of stroke, arterial or venous thromboembolism, severe hypertension, MI, hepatitis, benign or malignant hepatic neoplasm, pregnancy, breastfeeding, and estrogen-dependent breast neoplasm.

Relative contraindication: Dyslipidemia and undiagnosed vaginal bleeding.

Progestin-only Pills

It contains only synthetic progestin in low doses. Women having contraindications to estrogen-containing pills including heavy smokers, obesity, migraine with aura, past history of VTE, hypertension, and diabetes can use POPs. Progestin-only pills contain either LNG 30 μg, norethisterone 350 μg, desogestrel 75 μg, or drospirenone 4 mg.

Mechanism of Action

It involves thickening of cervical mucus and inhibition of ovulation. Pills are to be taken daily without any break. Desogestrel-containing pills have the greatest efficacy on ovulation inhibition. Due to its lack of association with VTE, stroke, and MI POPs can be safely used in perimenopausal women. Progestin-only pills do not affect bone marrow density or cause bone loss. Smokers can be advised to use POP.

Risk

There is no increased risk of breast cancer in POP users.

Noncontraceptive Benefits

Drospirenone-containing pills due to their antiandrogenic properties may have a better impact on arterial cardiovascular risk. Desogestrel pill may offer some benefits in the management of pain associated with endometriosis.

Disadvantage: Progestin-only pills cause a high risk of irregular bleeding or spotting and breakthrough bleeding. The newer option for POP drospirenone has higher amenorrhea rates.

Disadvantages of Progestin Only Pills

It includes an irregular bleeding pattern and a narrow window of safety for missed pills. A missed pill is one that is taken >3 hours late, or with desogestrel pills, >12 hours late.

Long-acting Reversible Contraception

It includes injectable contraceptions, implants, IUDs, and IUS.[4]

Injectable Contraception

Progestogen-only (1) DMPA; Depo-Provera and (2) recently licensed Sayana Press (medroxyprogesterone acetate 104 mg, given subcutaneously at 13-week intervals).

Progestogen-only

Depot medroxyprogesterone acetate (DMPA; Depo-Provera).

Dosing

It contains 150 mg of medroxyprogesterone acetate and its effect lasts for 3 months.

Mechanism of Action

Thickening of cervical mucus makes it impervious to sperm entry and ovulation suppression, and makes endometrium inhospitable to the ovum.

Side Effects

Irregular vaginal bleeding for first 3–6 months and amenorrhea after 6 months of use, weight gain, and osteopenia.

Noncontraceptive Benefit

May decrease menstrual cramps, reduce PMS and menorrhagia, protect against endometrial and ovarian cancer, helps to prevent uterine fibroid. Depot medroxyprogesterone acetate decreases benign breast disease, ovarian cysts and also reduces symptoms of endometriosis and the incidence of pelvic inflammatory disease (PID).

Special Consideration

The use of medroxyprogesterone acetate (MPA) reduces BMD by 5–6% in 5 years, with most loss happening in the first 2 years. Bone loss is reversible after cessation of injection DMPA, and bone mineral density recovers. Depot medroxyprogesterone acetate is a good contraceptive option for perimenopausal women as it reduces vasomotor symptoms, and effectively treats abnormal uterine bleeding and prevents endometrial hyperplasia. It reduces the risk of endometrial and ovarian cancer. Depot medroxyprogesterone acetate has a greater effect on lipids than other progestogen-only contraception methods and there is a theoretical risk of vascular disease in women with additional risk factors. Women without additional cardiovascular risk factors can use DMPA until the age of 50 years. There is limited data available about DMPA use in perimenopausal women and available studies suggest the use of DMPA is not associated with an increase in stroke, MI, or VTE.

Disadvantages

Weight gain of 1–2 kg after 1 year of DMPA use. There is little increased risk of cardiovascular disease associated with the use of DMPA.

Implant

The implant is a suitable method that can safely be used up until the age of 55 years.

Progestogen-only Implant

implanon—it is a subdermal implant; it releases 60 µg etonogestrel/day and is effective for 3 years. It is rapidly reversible contraception upon removal. It is a good option for women who dislike pills or IUDs. This implant should be fitted and removed, and trained by an operator. Unlike injectable contraceptive methods, this implant has no effect on bone mineral density. About 20% of women with this implant have amenorrhea. Women may experience unpredictable vaginal bleeding for the duration of use also the menstrual bleeding pattern is variable.

Special Considerations

Progestogen-only implant (IMP) is not associated with increased risks of VTE, stroke, or MI and has not been shown to affect bone mineral density (BMD). The IMP is the most effective form of contraception available with a 0.05% failure rate and there is no age restriction to its use. Nexplanon® IMP contains 68 mg of etonogestrel and is licensed for contraception for 3 years.

Noncontraceptive Benefits

The main noncontraceptive benefit of IMP is that it may alleviate menstrual and ovulatory pain.

Risks

The implant causes irregular bleeding in most women.

Intrauterine system is the most effective, long-acting reversible contraceptive method. It is a cost-effective contraceptive option for women that releases 20 μg LNG/day locally into the endometrium. Mirena or Levosert contains 52 mg of LNG and Jaydess contains 13.5 mg of LNG and is licensed for 3-year contraception.[5] Mirena releases 20 μg LNG per/day locally into the endometrium and its contraceptive effect is approved for 5 years of use. It can remain in place until the age of 55 years when natural cessation of fertility can be assumed for most women.[4]

Mechanism of Action: Progestin causes decidualization of the endometrium with thickening of cervical mucus and reduced tubal motility.

Benefits

Intrauterine system reduces menstrual blood loss by 40–50% and up to 80% in women with heavy menstrual bleeding (HMB).

Noncontraceptive Benefits

It can treat and prevent endometrial hyperplasia. Mirena is effective for reducing bleeding associated with fibroid, adenomyosis, and reducing symptoms of endometriosis.[2]

There is no evidence to support a link between breast cancer and IUS use, no risk of VTE or other systemic diseases, and no evidence of weight gain; hence, they are a safe option for perimenopausal women, especially those with HMB.

Jaydess has an insertion diameter smaller than the 52 mg IUS, so can be used in smaller uteri, nulliparous women, and older women in the later years of reproduction.

There is a 5% risk of expulsion in the first year and a 1 in 1,000 risk of uterine perforation. There is a small risk (<1 in 1,000) of infection.

Contraindications

Active cervical or pelvic infection and undiagnosed abnormal uterine bleeding.

Intrauterine Device

Copper T

It is the most effective method. Contraceptive effect of copper (Cu) T 380 A lasts for 10 years. Copper is spermicidal and makes endometrium hostile for implantation. It may cause slightly heavier menses in the first 3 months and expulsion up to 5% in the first year. When inserted in women older than 40 years they can be used until menopause. Intrauterine devices have minimal systemic effects so can be safely used in women with comorbidities that are more common in perimenopausal women.[2]

Sexually transmitted infections (STI) are not increased with Cu T. It can be inserted without gonococcal or chlamydial screening. No antibiotics are required after insertion. It can be used in women with a history of pelvic inflammatory disease.

Contraindications

Wilson disease, active cervical, or pelvic infection.

Natural family planning (NFP) methods become less reliable in perimenopause because of irregular menses. Ovulation becomes more difficult to predict and ovulation markers are difficult to interpret.

Withdrawal is a natural form of contraception. With lower fertility rates in perimenopause, withdrawal can be used as an adjunct to other methods, like NFP.

MALE AND FEMALE STERILIZATION

Sterilization (both male and female) is a suitable method and is the most commonly used method for couples in their 40s.[5] Male sterilization (vasectomy) has a lower failure rate 1 in 2,000 and a lower complication rate. The absence of sperm should be documented after the procedure. There is no increased risk of prostate or testes cancer.

Side Effects

Hematoma and infection.

Benefit

It is a safe method and there are no adverse health consequences.

Female Sterilization

It has a failure rate of 1 in 200. It involves occluding the fallopian tube which can be done either by laparoscopy or minilaparotomy or during cesarean.

Emergency Contraception

Options available are oral pills which are LNG or ulipristal acetate (UPA) and copper IUD. LNG EC contains 0.75 mg of LNG while UPA contains 30 mg. Effectiveness of EC decreases over time after the last sexual intercourse. Unlike Cu IUD, oral pills are only effective if taken prior to ovulation. Levonorgestrel can be used up to 72 hours after unprotected sexual intercourse (UPSI) UPA remains effective for up to 120 hours after UPSI. There is no age limit for using emergency contraception.

Copper IUD insertion needs to be done within 5 days after unprotected sex. It provides additional contraception for 10 years and it is much more effective than oral pills.

CONCLUSION

Contraception should be continued until menopause. All methods of contraception are available to perimenopausal women. Advice on contraception in older women depends on several issues including medical comorbidities and women's choices. There is no age restriction on the barrier method and it is the only way to protect against sexually shared infections. Combined hormonal contraceptives should be offered to women until 50 years if there is no health risk, e.g., smoking obesity high blood pressure. Combined oral contraceptives with 30 µg EE are first-line preparations due to lower risk of venous thromboembolism. Combined oral contraceptives have noncontraceptive benefits for menstrual complaints and also alleviate menopausal symptoms. Progestin only pill it is not associated with the risk of VTE stroke or MI and has not been shown to affect BMD. With injectable DMPA >50% of women become amenorrheic after 1 year of use and nearly 70% after 2 years of use. Unlike injectable contraceptive implants have no effect on BMD; however, may cause persistent and irregular bleeding. LNG IUS provides endometrial protection as part of heart and contraception and will need to be replaced every 5 years. The IUD is a safe and effective form of long-term contraception for period of 5–10 years. Sterilization is a nonreversible surgical procedure and all women considering sterilization must be counseled regarding the long-acting reversible contraception (LARC) method. Emergency contraception inhibits ovulation and is available in two forms EC pill and emergency IUD. Intrauterine device can remain in place for long-term contraception.

REFERENCES

1. Bakour SH, Hatti A, Whalen S. Contraceptive methods and issues around the menopause: an evidence update. Obstet Gynecol. 2017; 19(4):289-7.
2. Faculty of Sexual and Reproductive Healthcare Clinical Effectiveness Unit. FSRH clinical guidance: contraception for women over 40. London: FSRH; 2017 (Amended July 2023). https://www.fsrh.org/documents/fsrh-guidance-contraception-for-women-aged-over-40-years-2017/
3. Federation of Obstetric and Gynaecological Societies of India. Good Clinical Practice Recommendations (GCPR) on Combined Hormonal Contraceptives: Counselling and Use in Clinical Practice. [online] Available from: https://www.fogsi.org/wp-content/uploads/2015/11/CHC-GCPR-Final-version.pdf [Last accessed January, 2024].
4. National Collaborating Centre for Women's and Children's Health, National Institute for Health and Care Excellence. Long-acting reversible contraception: the effective and appropriate use of long-acting reversible contraception. London: RCOG Press; 2005.
5. British Menopause Society. Contraception for older women. [online] Available from: https://www.womens-health-concern.org/wp-content/uploads/2022/12/04-WHC-FACTSHEET-ContraceptionForTheOlderWoman-NOV22-B.pdf [Last accessed January, 2024].

CHAPTER 18

Contraception in Women with Abnormal Uterine Bleeding

Uma Wankhede, Swati Gurav

INTRODUCTION

Abnormal uterine bleeding (AUB) is defined as bleeding from the uterine corpus that is abnormal in regularity, volume, frequency, or duration and occurs in the absence of pregnancy. It can be acute or chronic. Acute AUB is defined as an episode of heavy bleeding that, in the opinion of the clinician, is of sufficient quantity to require immediate intervention to prevent further blood loss. Chronic AUB is defined as bleeding from the uterine corpus that is abnormal in volume, regularity, and/or timing that has been present for the majority of the last 6 months. Prevalence of AUB reported ranges from 11% to 24% intermenstrual bleeding (IMB), postcoital bleeding (PCB), heavy menstrual bleeding (HMB), and postmenopausal bleeding (PMB) are causes of AUB. AUB impairs women's quality of life and also raises concern about gynecological cancers. The National Institute for Health and Clinical Excellence (NICE) defines HMB as excessive menstrual blood loss which interferes with the woman's physical, emotional, social, and material quality of life.

PAST, PRESENT, AND FUTURE

The International Federation of Gynecology and Obstetrics (FIGO) introduced a classification system for the causes of AUB in 2011 known by the acronym PALM-COEIN (Polyp; Adenomyosis; Leiomyoma; Malignancy and Hyperplasia; Coagulopathy; Ovulatory Disorders; Endometrial factors; Iatrogenic; and Not classified).

The etiology of AUB is classified as structural (PALM) and nonstructural (COEIN) causes for a woman's menstrual irregularities. PMB, IMB, and PCB could be symptoms of gynecological malignancies such as cervical and endometrial cancer. The FIGO also defined normal and abnormal limits for menstrual parameters.[1]

DIAGNOSIS OF ABNORMAL UTERINE BLEEDING

Thorough history, focused on menstrual bleeding details about duration and regularity of cycle, and physical examination guide about further investigations, diagnosis, and management. Pregnancy needs to be excluded. Examination includes abdominal and pelvic examination of the vulva, vagina, and cervix using a speculum; structural and nonstructural causes are explored from initial assessment. Laboratory evaluation depends on clinical presentation, including complete blood count, targeted screening for bleeding disorder, hormonal assessment, and pelvic imaging. Urgent pelvic ultrasound may be needed if any associated symptom such as pain or suspicious clinical finding of pregnancy or malignancy. Evaluation is done in acute AUB to rule out trauma along with exploration of cause and initial management involves stabilization with treatment of cause. Endometrial tissue sampling needs to be performed in patients with AUB who are older than 40 years as a first-line test. Endometrial sampling also should be performed in patients younger than 40 years with a history of unopposed estrogen exposure (such as seen in patients with obesity or polycystic ovary syndrome, diabetes, family history of ovarian, and endometrial malignancy) unresponsive to medical management and persistent AUB.

MANAGEMENT OF ABNORMAL UTERINE BLEEDING

Management depends on clinical assessment for cause of bleeding and women's desire for contraception. Combined oral contraceptives (COCs) and oral progestins taken in multidose regimens also are commonly used for acute AUB. For chronic AUB, treatment is targeted to underlying structural or medical cause explored after clinical assessment. It consists of (1) balancing prostaglandin E2 (PGE2)/prostaglandin F2 alpha (PGF2-alpha) levels, (2) use of antifibrinolytic to arrest bleeding, (3) controlling endometrial growth and arrest endometrial sloughing by using combined hormonal contraceptives (CHCs) (pill, patch, and ring), (4) suppression of endometrial growth and provides lighter, predictable bleeding—progestin-only contraceptive methods (progesterone-only pill, implants, injectables, or an intrauterine system) reduce menstrual blood loss but may induce amenorrhea over long-term use.

ABNORMAL BLEEDING IN WOMEN USING CONTRACEPTION

Abnormal bleeding pattern can occur within the first 3 months of use of any new hormonal preparation such as contraceptive pill, injectable contraceptive, progestin-containing contraceptives, or levonorgestrel (LNG) intrauterine device (IUD). However, if this abnormal bleeding is persistent, it can be distressing for patient, leading to noncompliance. Details of history regarding compliance of pill and timing of pill intake and also any drug intake interfering with pill need to be explored. Women with irregular bleeding are advised to continue same contraceptive for 3 months and usually bleeding settles with time of 3–6 months. Irregular bleeding is frequent and common with progestin-only contraceptives. Women using hormonal contraceptives who have abnormal problematic bleeding assessment should go through history excluding sexually transmitted infection (STI) and underlying pathology (structural, neoplasia, polyp, etc.), checking cervical screening and ruling out pregnancy. Regimens such as estrogen supplementation or tranexamic acid may help to reduce bleeding induced by progestogen-only contraceptives. 70% of women achieve amenorrhea who are on progestogen-only contraception (progesterone-only pill, implants, injectables, or an intrauterine system) for long term. Also, breakthrough bleeding most commonly occurs, induced by progestogen-only contraceptives within the first 6 months and is the main reason for noncompliance of method of contraception.[2]

CONTRACEPTION AND ABNORMAL UTERINE BLEEDING

An individual approach should be taken while considering contraception for women with AUB. Excluding underlying pathology, pregnancy as well as sexually shared infections are key elements. In patients with idiopathic AUB and wish to have effective contraception, LNG-releasing intrauterine system (LNG-IUS) is recommended as first-line therapy to reduce menstrual bleeding. In patients with AUB desirous of continued fertility, in whom LNG-IUS are contraindicated, use of COCs are recommended as second-line therapy. Based on etiology in AUB-malignancy (AUB-M) with endometrial hyperplasia (EH) with atypia, hysterectomy is the standard treatment. In AUB-M with EH without atypia, LNG-IUS can be considered as first-line therapy.

BARRIER METHODS

Male condom: When male condoms are used correctly and consistently, failure rate is 2%. Condoms are also used as part of dual protection for STI risk reduction. It can be used by male partners of women with AUB. Most of male condoms are made of latex. Latex allergy is found in 2–4% of general population, who can use synthetic plastic isoprene condoms or lamb cecum condoms.

Female condoms: It can also reduce STI risk. They are best used by women whose partners are not using male condoms. It fits loosely inside vagina and covers perineum. Female condoms are expensive and have higher failure rates, so research is needed to reduce cost.

Diaphragms: These are made up of latex rubber and must be used along with spermicide nonoxynol-9 gel left in place for 6 hours after intercourse. It prevents passage of sperm into cervical canal.

Natural family planning methods: These include withdrawal, fertility awareness, and lactational amenorrhea. It works only when cycles are regular (26–32 days). For these methods to be effective, counting of fertile days is important. In women with AUB, prediction of ovulation and fertile period can be difficult precluding use of these methods.

EMERGENCY CONTRACEPTION

Emergency contraception is method of postcoital pregnancy prevention. There are two forms available (1) emergency contraceptive pill, (2) IUD.

Most effective method with failure rate of 1 in 1,000 is IUD to be fitted within 5 days of coitus. LNG and ulipristal acetate (UPA) pills work by suppressing ovulation up to beginning of luteinizing hormone (LH) surge, prior to ovulation. It can be option for women with infrequent sex and AUB to prevent unwanted pregnancy and starting regular, suitable hormonal contraception afterward.

Sterilization

Female sterilization is more common nonreversible surgical procedure, even though vasectomy is a safer permanent male sterilization procedure. Different techniques have been used for tubal occlusion. Pomeroy method of tubal ligation is preferred to perform soon after delivery. Tubal ligation can be performed as interval technique by laparoscopy or minilaparotomy procedure. In patients with AUB, desirous of contraception as permanent method, sterilization can be considered.

Combined Hormonal Contraceptives

The CHCs have both estrogen and a progestin to provide cycle control. There are different hormonal formulations, different regimens, and different doses. In addition to pill, the transdermal patch and vaginal ring are other options. The primary mechanisms of action of all CHCs are to thicken cervical mucus and suppress ovulation. Traditionally, combination birth control pills were given in packets with 21 active pills and 7 placebo pills to provide monthly scheduled bleeding.

Risks

Health risk attributed to use of CHCs include increase in both venous and arterial thrombosis, resulting in pulmonary embolism, myocardial infarction (MI), and stroke. Melasma (facial pigmentation) is seen as a result of estrogen-containing contraceptive use. Other side effects with oral contraceptive use include headaches, breast tenderness, weight gain, mood changes, and gastrointestinal upsets.

The contraceptive patch and the vaginal ring were developed to eliminate requirement of daily administration. Both patches and the ring are designed to be used for 3 weeks and stopped for 1 week to induce scheduled bleeding.

One of the treatment option for chronic AUB is medroxyprogesterone acetate (MPA) 10 mg tablet orally each day for last 10 days of cycle, estrogen-containing oral contraceptive pills, transdermal patches, or vaginal rings. The best treatment options for anovulatory AUB to arrest endometrial growth resulting in lighter predictable bleeding are estrogen-containing oral contraceptive pills, transdermal patches, or vaginal rings. Extended cycle use of oral contraceptives or uninterrupted use of vaginal contraceptive rings for 3–12 months can also prevent scheduled bleeding for substantial periods of time.

Combined Oral Contraceptive Pill

Oral contraceptive pills suppress pituitary gonadotropin release, thus inhibiting ovulation and causing endometrial atrophy. COC pill is useful in reducing menstrual blood loss and establishing regular cycles. Advantages of the COC pills are reduction of dysmenorrhea and providing contraception.

Noncontraceptive health benefits include treatment of acne. These methods also significantly reduce the risk of endometrial and ovarian cancer. Extended-cycle products provide distinct benefits to women with menstrual discomfort, dysmenorrhea, and menorrhagia. Extended cycle contraceptive pill is useful treatment option in chronic AUB causing endometrial suppression resulting in lighter bleeding or to create amenorrhea.

It is available as monophasic and quadraphasic pills. It can be used for 3–6 months (spontaneous relief thereafter) These should be avoided in women with thrombosis or a family history of idiopathic venous thromboembolism (VTE) The most common side effects include weight gain, abdominal discomfort, and midcycle breakthrough bleeding.

Combined oral contraceptive pills are preferred treatment option for women with AUB where etiology is leiomyoma, COEIN in PALM–COEIN etiology, or AUB-ovulatory dysfunction (AUB-O). One of the therapeutic option for acute heavy uterine bleeding is oral contraceptive pill with 35 μg of ethinyl estradiol (EE), 1.0 mg of norethindrone acetate, one tablet orally every 8 hours for 7 days, then 20 μg of EE, 1.0 mg of norethindrone acetate pills, one tablet orally once daily for 21 days.

Progestin-only contraceptives: Injected or implanted progestogen prevents proliferation of the endometrium depot intramuscular injections given 3 monthly. In cases of AUB on injection or implant users, bleeding is likely to stop completely.

Medroxyprogesterone acetate (Depo-Provera) is useful treatment option in chronic AUB causing endometrial suppression resulting in lighter bleeding or to create amenorrhea. LNG-IUS 20 μg/24 hours and depot MPA (DMPA) injections induce complete amenorrhea in a significant percentage of women with longer use and is very effective treatment option in AUB.

Progestogen-only pill (POP): Formulations either include desogestrel (DSG), norethisterone, or LNG. Women using a DSG pill are more likely to become anovulatory than women using traditional preparations (97% of DSG users vs. 60% of LNG users). POP can be used until the age at which natural loss of fertility is assumed. POPs do not cause blood pressure to increase, their effect on lipid profiles and diabetes is minimal. POP is not associated with increased risks of VTE, stroke, or MI and has not been shown to affect bone mineral density (BMD). They are safe for use in women suffering from migraine.

Risks

There is a small increased risk of breast cancer in women who take POPs, but this risk is reduced when the user stops taking pills. POP can be used in smokers over the age of 35 years.

Noncontraceptive benefits: DSG pill can have benefits in the management of pain associated with endometriosis, menstruation, and ovulation as it suppresses ovulation in most women.

Cyclic oral progestins (from day 5 to 26) are recommended if COCs are contraindicated in AUB-COEIN etiology.

Depot MPA is an injectable contraceptive administered every 3 months. One of the side effects is amenorrhea. The NICE guideline indicated that up to 47% of women receiving DMPA (100–150 mg) had amenorrhea at 1-year follow-up. It does not have impact on future fertility; it is long lasting and effective and can be used where estrogen use is contraindicated. Common side effects can include irregular bleeding, weight gain, amenorrhea, and premenstrual-like syndrome. Less common effects include revisable loss of BMD.[3]

One of the therapeutic options for acute heavy uterine bleeding is MPA 20 mg orally every 8 hours for 3 days with intramuscular injection of DMPA 150 mg.

Implant

Contraceptive implant reduces blood loss; however, LNG-IUS is most effective treatment option in AUB.

Progestogen-only implant: It is a 4 cm × 2 mm rod which is implanted in the inner aspect of the upper arm, usually on the nondominant side. This is the most effective reversible method of contraception with immediate return of fertility on removal and can be used for up to 3 years. This implant needs to be fitted and removed by a trained operator. There is no user failure rate, but additional contraceptive protection is advised if not fitted within the first 5 days of menstruation. Unlike injectable contraceptive methods, this implant has no effect on BMD.

LNG-IUS: It is medicated IUDs which release LNG which reduce menstrual blood loss by up to 90% in women with menorrhagia with increasing effectiveness after approximately 6 months of use. LNG-IUS is more effective at reducing menstrual blood loss than any other hormonal preparations for AUB (COC, oral progestogens, tranexamic acid, mefenamic acid, and flurbiprofen). Studies reported similar outcomes of pictorial blood loss between LNG-IUS and endometrial ablation after 24 months follow-up. LNG-IUS is the most cost-effective means of reducing menstrual blood loss in women with HMB compared with pharmacological therapies and is also an effective contraceptive.

- Its main advantages are relief of dysmenorrhea, effective contraception, and long-term control of menorrhagia after insertion.

- Side effects reported are IMB and breast tenderness in the first few months following insertion.
- Contraindicated in pregnancy, unexplained vaginal bleeding, and uterine sepsis.

In AUB-O, if COCs are contraindicated or patient is unwilling for COCs, LNG-IUS is recommended if she wishes to use it for at least one year. For AUB due to polyp, hysteroscopic surgical removal is suggested. In cases of multiple polyps or polypoidal endometrium and fertility is not desired, it is suggested to perform hysteroscopic polypectomy followed by LNG-IUS insertion after confirmation of benign lesion on histopathology. In AUB cases due to adenomyosis (AUB-A) willing for contraception, LNG-IUS is recommended as first-line therapy. For intramural or submucosal myoma, treatment options are individualized depending on age, parity, and contraception and fertility desires. Women with intramural or submucosal myoma willing for contraception can be medically managed with LNG-IUS if other medical treatment fails and patient is not trying to conceive for at least one year. For intramural myoma <4 cm diameter in women above 40 years of age, not desirous of continued fertility, hysterectomy is the definitive treatment; however, medical management including LNG-IUS may be tried. In AUB-M with EH without atypia, LNG-IUS can be considered as first-line therapy; oral progestins can be used if LNG-IUS is contraindicated or if patient is unwilling for LNG-IUS. In patients with AUB-coagulopathy (AUB-C), nonhormonal treatment with tranexamic acid as primary option and hormonal treatment with COCs/LNG-IUS as secondary option are recommended in consultation with a hematologist.

In AUB-M with endometrial malignancy, standard protocol for management of malignancy should be followed. EH is caused by unopposed increase in estrogen upon the endometrium, and therefore risk factors include raised body mass index (BMI), anovulation driven by perimenopause and polycystic ovary syndrome (PCOS), nulliparity, estrogen-secreting tumors, and drug-induced causes such as hormone replacement therapy (HRT) and tamoxifen use. In AUB-M with EH with atypia, hysterectomy is the standard treatment. Most cases of EH without atypia regress during follow-up period. Risk factors such as obesity, diabetes, etc. need to be managed and follow-up with biannual endometrial biopsy is considered. LNG-IUS has higher regression rate and also effective in reducing menstrual blood loss. Surgical management for hysterectomy is considered only if not responding to hormonal treatment after 6–12 months or progression to atypical hyperplasia during follow-up.

In patients with AUB-coagulopathy (AUB-C), nonhormonal treatment with tranexamic acid as primary option and hormonal treatment with COCs/LNG-IUS as secondary option are recommended in consultation with a hematologist.

Centchroman is an option when steroidal hormones and other medical options are not suitable.

Intrauterine contraceptive device (IUCD) containing copper is not a preferred option in AUB as it may contribute to IMB and HMB.

CONCLUSION

Treatment options for management of acute and chronic AUB depend on etiology, clinical evaluation, and exploring underlying cause. Pregnancy, STI, and malignancy need to be excluded in all cases. Detailed history is explored about bleeding pattern, cycle length, and regularity. Regarding ongoing contraceptive use, while for oral hormonal contraceptive pills, its compliance and missed pill need to be explored. LNG-IUS is considered as first-line treatment for AUB due to adenomyosis, selected cases of leiomyoma, and EH without atypia and COEIN causes in PALM–COEIN etiology of AUB.[4]

Its main advantages are relief of dysmenorrhea, effective contraception, and long-term control of menorrhagia following insertion.

Side effects reported are IMB and breast tenderness in the first few months following insertion.

Combined oral contraceptives are first-line treatment option for women in AUB-O willing for contraception. COC are offered to women with intramural or subserosal myomas desirous of preserving fertility as second-line therapy. COC can be offered for symptomatic relief in AUB-A where LNG-IUS and gonadotropin hormone-releasing hormone (GnRH) agonists cannot be indicated. In AUB-COEIN etiology, COCs are recommended as second-line therapy in patients desiring effective contraception but unwilling or unsuitable for LNG-IUS.

REFERENCES

1. The Royal College of Obstetricians and Gynaecologists. (2009). Management of Unscheduled Bleeding in Women Using Hormonal Contraception. [online] Available from: https://www.rcog.org.uk/guidance/browse-all-guidance/other-guidelines-and-reports/management-of-unscheduled-bleeding-in-women-using-hormonal-contraception/ [Last accessed January, 2024].
2. American College of Obstetricians and Gynecologists. ACOG committee opinion no. 557: Management of acute abnormal uterine bleeding in nonpregnant reproductive aged women. Obstet Gynecol. 2013;121(4): 891-6.
3. National Collaborating Centre for Women's and Children's Health (UK). Heavy Menstrual Bleeding. London: RCOG Press; 2007.
4. The Royal College of Obstetricians and Gynaecologists. (2016). Management of endometrial hyperplasia, green top guideline No. 67. [online] Available from: https://www.rcog.org.uk/guidance/browse-all-guidance/green-top-guidelines/management-of-endometrial-hyperplasia-green-top-guideline-no-67/ [Last accessed January, 2024].

CHAPTER 19

Contraception in Special Situation—Acne and Hirsutism

Sangeeta Tajpuriya

INTRODUCTION

Acne and hirsutism are the manifestation of hyperandrogenemia. Women seeking contraception with acne and hirsutism need tailored approach to combat the androgenic features. The presence of terminal hair in androgenic pattern on the face is known as "hirsutism". Acne is colonization of dead epithelial cells and sebum by the bacterium *Propionibacterium* acnes. If left untreated it, the inflammation leads to the development of papules, pustules, and nodules. The metabolic disorder associated with hyperandrogenemia is polycystic ovary syndrome (PCOS). Acne, hirsutism, and virilization are the most common features of PCOS. A woman with features of hyperandrogenemia, if counseled and informed about the dual nature of combined oral contraceptive in which along with contraceptive added advantage of antiandrogenic activity is available, would be more than willing to use the prescribed oral contraceptives.

PAST, PRESENT, AND FUTURE

Since the advent of "combined oral contraceptive," though the formulation contains both the estrogen and progesterone component, it is mainly the progesterone component which is the main determining factor.[1]

- Progesterone component does the contraceptive role by inhibiting preovulatory luteinizing hormone (LH)-surge which suppresses ovulation and making cervical mucus thick, so it becomes impermeable to sperm penetration.
- Estrogen component helps in cycle control and aids in ovarian suppression.

Past

Progestational agents after being metabolized in the body have different biological effect on different organs of the body. Some have estrogenic, some antiestrogenic, and some have more androgenic effects.

According to the derivatives of progesterone component, the pills were categorized into different generation pills.

First-generation Pill

Norethisterone-containing pills are called first-generation pills.

These progestational compounds have moderate androgen activity.

Second-generation Pill

Levonorgestrel is the progestational agent of the second-generation pill. It has strong progestational and androgenic effects than the first-generation pills.

Present

Third-generation Pill

Friendly progesterone derivatives were derived from 19-nortestosterone derivatives as *gestodene, desogestrel,* and *norgestimate.* Each of the derivatives mimics natural progestational features, by binding specifically to progesterone receptors and exhibiting strong antiestrogenic and minimal to absolutely no androgenic effects.

Drospironone is derived from 17-alpha-spironolactone; an analog of spironolactone. It has antimineral corticoid and strong antiandrogenic properties.

Cyproterone acetate is the progestin with the highest antiandrogenic activity and is used to treat various androgen-dependent conditions.

Oral contraceptive (OC) pills containing spironolactone, gestodene, desogestrel, and cyproterone acetate are called third-generation pills.

TREATMENT

Contraception in women having features of hyperandrogenemia should be targeted on decreasing free androgen levels.

Ovarian steroid production inhibition can be achieved by administering estrogen and progesterone together in the form of oral contraceptives with progestogens having strong antiandrogenic activity. Hence, third-generation OC pills are the treatment of choice.[2]

Adrenal androgens production is also decreased by this formulation. They also inhibit 5-α-reductase activity in androgen peripheral target structures.

Treatment should last for at least 6 months as new generation OC pills will slow the growth of new terminal hairs and not the existing hair follicle.

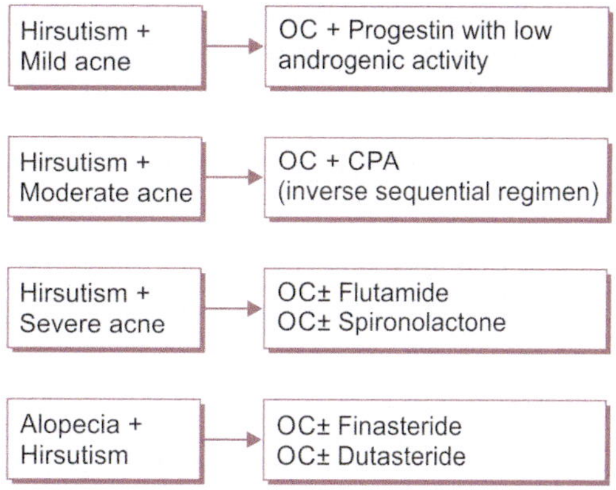

Fig. 1: Treatment of hirsutism with oral contraceptives (OCs) and widely used antiandrogens.[4]

Strong antiandrogen agents such as *flutamide and finasteride* are to be taken into consideration in some nonresponsive hyperandrogenemia group. Flutamide acts by blocking androgen receptors[3] and finasteride acts by inhibiting 5-α-reductase intracellular enzyme activity. These two agents are combined with new generation OC pills to reinforce the contraceptive effects in this special hyperandrogenemia, hirsutism, and acne group.

Oral Contraceptive Pills

- Ethinyloestradiol 30 μg + DRSP 3 mg
- Ethinyloestradiol 35 μg + CPA 2 mg.

Inverse Sequential Regimen

12.5, 25, or 50 mg CPA + 20–30 μg ethinylestradiol (EE) is the reverse sequential regimen.

Various treatment modalities to prescribe OC pills with antiandrogen agents are shown in **Figure 1** above.

REFERENCES

1. Spielberg TC, Rories C, Rejman JJ, Goldberger A, Fink K, Lau CK, et al. Steroid action on gene

expression: possible roles of regulatory genes and nuclear receptor sites. Biol Reprod. 1989; 40(1):54-69.

2. De Leo V, Morgante G, Piomboni P, Musacchio MC, Petraglia F, Cianci A. Evaluation of effects of an oral contraceptive containing ethinyl estradiol combined with drospirenone on adrenal steroidogenesis in hyperandrogenic women with polycystic ovary syndrome. Fertil Steril. 2007;8:113-7.
3. De Leo V, Fulghesu AM, La Marca A, Morgante G, Pasqui L, Talluri B, et al. Hormonal and clinical effects of GnRH agonist alone, or in combination with a combined oral contraceptive or flutamide in women with severe hirsutism. Gynecol Endocrinol. 2000; 14:411-6.
4. De Leo V, Musacchio MC, Cappelli V, Piomboni P, Morgante G. Hormonal contraceptives: pharmacology tailored to women's health. Hum Reprod Update. 2016; 22(5):634-46.

CHAPTER 20

Guidelines for Use of Contraceptives in Human Immunodeficiency Virus and Sexually Transmitted Diseases

Ashish Kale, Sushma Sharma, Jaya Barla

INTRODUCTION

The rights and wellbeing of women and teenage girls depend critically on their ability to access sexual and reproductive health services and information, including a wide variety of contraceptive options.[1-4] Numerous hormonal and nonhormonal modern contraception methods offer important advantages for both personal and societal health. The World Health Organization (WHO) places a high priority on the creation and upkeep of current, evidence-based recommendations about the safety of contraceptives for people with certain medical disorders or other characteristics that are relevant from a medical standpoint.[5]

MEDICAL ELIGIBILITY CRITERIA

An extensive set of recommendations on the medical safety of contraceptive methods is furnished by the medical eligibility criteria (MEC) for contraceptive use (the MEC), 5th edition, to national policymakers and family planning programs. This facilitates the informed development of national policies, protocols, and programs.[5] The removal of pointless medical hurdles to contraception is facilitated by global recommendations on medical safety and eligibility.

Countries have been utilizing the MEC for >20 years to increase safety and raise the standard of care provided for contraception. With the help of ongoing monitoring and evaluations of published research, safety guidance is kept current. WHO published the 5th edition of the MEC in 2015.[5] In the context of >80 medical illnesses or personally relevant medical traits, this edition includes >2,000 recommendations for 25 various contraceptive techniques. Depending on the person, more than one requirement may need to be taken into account while selecting a contraceptive method.[5]

The MECs recommendations are based on a number of factors, such as whether using a contraceptive technique worsens the medical condition or poses extra health risks, and whether it would be in the best interest of the patient. The MECs recommendations are based on a number of factors, such as whether using a contraceptive technique worsens an existing medical condition, poses new health risks, or reduces the effectiveness of the method due to the condition.[5]

In light of recent research, the WHO updated its recommendations for using contraceptives to reflect the fact that women who are at high risk for contracting HIV can use any reversible method of birth control, including intrauterine devices (IUDs), implants, and injectable progestogen-only products, without an increased risk of contracting HIV.

The independent Guideline Development Group, which was assembled to provide information to WHO, reviewed the most recent research in order to update its recommendations for the WHO guideline, MEC for contraceptive usage. In addition to doing a systematic analysis of all available data on copper-bearing IUDs and human immunodeficiency virus (HIV) risk, this group evaluated all research on hormonal contraception and the risk of contracting HIV that has been published since the previous review, which was released in 2016.

Sub-Saharan Africa, which has the highest rates of HIV transmission but also some of the biggest obstacles to ensuring women have access to a full range of contraceptive alternatives, is particularly affected by the worldwide recommendations. Currently, just 24% of African women aged 15–49 years who desire to put off or avoid having children have easy access to contemporary contraception. Across all WHO areas, this is the demand that is least addressed.

CONSIDERING THE FACTS

The ECHO experiment, a randomized clinical trial that found no statistically significant differences in HIV acquisition among women using intramuscular depot medroxyprogesterone acetate (DMPA-IM), copper IUDs, or levonorgestrel (LNG) implants, served as the foundation for much of the recent research. The observational studies' low to low-moderate quality evidence that was previously available to support WHO's recommendations have been replaced by this new and high-quality research.[6]

SEXUALLY TRANSMITTED INFECTION PREVENTION EDUCATION IN THE PERSPECTIVE OF CONTRACEPTIVE SERVICES

The ECHO study,[7] which was conducted in Eswatini, Kenya, South Africa, and Zambia in communities where HIV prevalence was expected to be high, also showed alarmingly high rates of HIV acquisition and other sexually transmitted infections (STIs) among women seeking contraceptive services, particularly younger women, regardless of which of the three contraceptive methods they used.

It is imperative to give women access to high-quality HIV and STI prevention and testing services as well as a variety of contraception methods that are compatible with their values, preferences, opinions, and concerns. These may include partner testing, condom marketing, preexposure prophylaxis (PrEP), connections to antiretroviral therapy for those testing HIV-positive, and PrEP in areas with high HIV prevalence.

To assist the implementation of these updated recommendations, WHO will collaborate with Ministries of Health, other organizations offering contraceptive and STI/HIV services, and civil society, especially youth organizations. In order to ensure that their perspectives are heard and taken into account across WHO in connection to HIV and sexual and reproductive health and rights, WHO has established an advisory committee of women living with HIV.

THE FOUR-CATEGORY SCALE[8]

In order to establish medical eligibility for use of each contraceptive method in the context of specific health issues or dangers **(Table 1)**, the MEC for Contraceptive Use guideline has adopted a four-category scale since 1996. (Such as women at high risk of HIV).

Contraceptive techniques are divided into one of four numbered groups for each condition or trait:

1. A circumstance for which the use of a contraceptive technique is not prohibited.

2. A circumstance in which the benefits of utilizing the approach typically outweigh the theoretical or shown risks, although further thought and counseling may be required when selecting this way.
3. A circumstance where the benefits of employing the technique typically surpass the theoretical or verified risks.
4. A situation that poses an unacceptably high risk to one's health if the contraceptive method is applied.

Progestogen-only injectable contraception was classified as category 2 in 2016 based on the low to low-moderate evidence that was available at the time, with special consideration being advised for women who were at high risk of HIV. Due to the change from category 1 to 2, progestogen-only injectable contraception is no longer thought to have harmful health effects for women who are at high risk of HIV.

TABLE 1: Medical eligibility criteria (MEC) categories for contraceptive eligibility.

1. A condition for which there is no restriction for the use of the contraceptive method
2. A condition where the advantages of using the method generally outweigh the theoretical or proven risks
3. A condition where the theoretical or proven risks usually outweigh the advantages of using the method
4. A condition which represents an unacceptable health risk if the contraceptive method is used

Table 2 displays the practical interpretation and implementation of the categories.

RECOMMENDATIONS FOR WOMEN AT HIGH RISK OF HIV INFECTION TO CONSIDER CONTRACEPTION

The MEC for Contraceptive Use[5] for Women at High Risk of HIV currently classify all hormonal contraceptive methods and IUDs into Category 1. As a result, women who are highly susceptible to HIV are encouraged to use any type of contraception.

1. All progestogen-only contraceptive methods, including progestogen-only pills (POPs), intramuscular depot medroxyprogesterone acetate (DMPA-IM), subcutaneous DMPA (DMPA-SC), norethisterone enanthate (NET-EN) injectables, LNG implants, and etonogestrel implants, are permissible for use without restriction by women at high risk.
2. Copper-bearing IUDs (Cu-IUDs) and LNG-IUDs can be used without limitation by women who are highly susceptible to contracting HIV (MEC Category 1). Many women at high risk for HIV are also at high risk for other STIs, so providers should take this into consideration when considering the use of IUDs. For these

TABLE 2: Illustrating the medical eligibility criteria (MEC) categories and how they are applied.

Category	*With goods resources for clinical judgment*	*With limited resources for clinical judgment*
1.	Use the method in any circumstances	Yes, use the method
2.	Generally use the method	
3.	Use of the method not usually recommended unless more appropriate methods are not available or not acceptable	No, do not use the method
4.	Method not to be used	

women, they should consult the MEC recommendation on women at increased risk of STIs and the selected practice recommendations for contraceptive use on STI screening before IUD insertion.[5,9]

3. All combined hormonal contraceptive methods, including combined oral contraceptives (COCs), combined injectable contraceptives (CICs), combined contraceptive patches (P), and combined vaginal rings, are permissible for use by women at a high risk of HIV infection (MEC Category 1) (CVR).

REFERENCES

1. World Health Organization. Ensuring human rights in the provision of contraceptive information and services: guidance and recommendations. Geneva: World Health Organization; 2014.
2. World Health Organization. Framework for ensuring human rights in the provision of contraceptive information and services. Geneva: World Health Organization; 2014.
3. World Health Organization. The thirteenth general programme of work, 2019–2023: promote health, keep the world safe, serve the vulnerable. Geneva: World Health Organization; 2019.
4. World Health Organization. Reproductive health strategy to accelerate progress towards the attainment of international development goals and targets. Geneva: World Health Organization; 2004.
5. World Health Organization. Medical eligibility criteria for contraceptive use, fifth edition. Geneva: World Health Organization; 2015.
6. World Health Organization. (2019). WHO revises recommendations on hormonal contraceptive use for women at high HIV risk. [online] Available from https://www.who.int/news/item/29-08-2019-who-revises-recommendations-on-hormonal-contraceptive-use-for-women-at-high-hiv-risk [Last accessed November, 2019].
7. World Health Organization. Actions for improved clinical and prevention services and choices: preventing HIV and other sexually transmitted infections among women and girls using contraceptive services in contexts with high HIV incidence, June 2020: policy brief. Geneva: World Health Organization; 2020.
8. Folger SG, Curtis KM, Tepper NK, Gaffield ME, Marchbanks PA. Guidance on medical eligibility criteria for contraceptive use: identification of research gaps. Contraception. 2010;82(1):113-8.
9. World Health Organization. Selected practice recommendations for contraceptive use: third edition. Geneva: World Health Organization; 2016

CHAPTER 21

Contraception after Abortion

Ashish Kale, Sushma Sharma

INTRODUCTION AND BACKGROUND

Postabortion family planning/use of contraceptive methods is the counseling for the adoption and implementation of contraceptive methods at the time of clinically managing an abortion or before the return of fertility in the postabortion period.[1] The World Health Organization has estimated that world over, around 210 million women become pregnant every year. Out of these 250 million, 75 million pregnancies end up with a negative outcome as either abortions (induced or spontaneous) or stillbirths.[2] Majority of these women do not desire to become pregnant again in the near future. It is also recommended by the World Health Organization (WHO) to ideally allow a time period space of at least 6 months to lapse between an abortion and the next conception. Hence, it is important to offer family planning services as a part of postabortion care. Doing this can improve not just contraceptive acceptance, but will help in breaking the undesirable cycle of repeated unwanted pregnancies.[3,4]

It is seen that women coming for abortion services to a facility rarely come back to the same center to seek family planning services even though they do not want to conceive again in the immediate future. This fact reiterates the need for immediate selection of the postabortion period as the opportune time to provide contraceptive advice and services, when the woman is still at the abortion care facility or in while she is in contact with the healthcare provider.

COUNSELING REGARDING POSTABORTION CONTRACEPTION: A CRITICAL COMPONENT

Counseling is perhaps the most crucial and result-deciding component in providing quality postabortion family planning services—the timing of which is ideally before the management of abortion, enabling the couple to choose a method that may be brought into the effective concomitantly.

ELIGIBILITY CRITERIA FOR POSTABORTION FAMILY PLANNING/CONTRACEPTION METHODS

Prior to selecting to offer any family planning method to a woman in the postabortion period, it is crucial to establish:

- There have been no severe complications of abortion which she has undergone and she does not need any further management for the same.
- The couples should receive a detailed informed choice of the various suitable

methods of contraception, should be counseled thoroughly in the postabortion period, and give informed consent for the selected method of family planning.

- Once a particular family planning method has been selected, the healthcare provider should screen the woman for eligibility for the selected method.

TIME OF INITIATION OF CONTRACEPTIVE METHODS AFTER ABORTION

See **Table 1**.

POSTABORTION INTRAUTERINE COPPER DEVICE[5]

The healthcare provider offering the abortion services should ensure that the woman seeking an abortion has been provided with adequate information and counseling during postabortion period. The woman should be able to make an informed choice prior to intrauterine copper device (IUCD) insertion. Copper (Cu) IUCD 380 A/Cu IUCD 375, which provides contraception for 10 years/ 5 years respectively, can be inserted as per the informed choice and preference of the patient.

Eligibility Criteria

See **Table 2**.

Clinical Evaluation and Eligibility Screening of the Patient

Evaluation and fitness for immediate postabortion IUCD is done in a manner consisting of two phases:

1. The first assessment is done in order to review the woman's general, medical, reproductive, contraceptive, and obstetric history. This first assessment also checks her eligibility for the method along with preprocedure evaluation for the IUCD insertion.
2. The patient's second assessment is done in the time just prior to insertion of the IUCD. This assessment is done to rule out current genital tract infections or the risk of infection. It also checks for any abnormal hemorrhage and genital tract injury.

Clinical Technique of Postabortion Intrauterine Copper Device Insertion

See **Table 3**.

Follow-up Advice after Intrauterine Copper Device Insertion

- Before the woman leaves the healthcare facility, she should be advised to:
    - Revisit the center for postabortion follow-up within 1–2 weeks for:
        - Clinical evaluation of her physical condition,
        - Ruling out any possibility of failure of abortion and continuation of the pregnancy. To rule out sepsis and incomplete abortion
        - To identify any immediate complications due to the IUCD insertion itself.
    - Plan and fix a date for a visit again as a routine follow-up of IUCD after 1 month, preferably after the next menstrual cycle.
    - Immediately visit the center and report as an emergency if any warning signs/symptoms appear.
- Follow-up care and management of any issues related to postabortion IUCD should be similar to that of interval IUCD.

TABLE 1: Time of initiation of contraceptive methods after abortion.

	Family planning method	***Time of initiation after abortion***
Following first-trimester abortion		
Spontaneous abortion on vacuum aspiration (for incomplete/ induced abortion)	Combined oral contraceptive pills—mono-/bi-/triphasic	Can be initiated with *immediate effect*
	Progestin-only contraceptive pills	Can be initiated with *immediate effect*
	Centchroman pills/Saheli	Can be initiated with *immediate effect*
	Injectable progesterone—injection DMPA	Can be initiated with *immediate effect*
	Condoms	Can be used with *immediate effect* by the male partner
	IUCD	• If there are no signs of genital tract infection/ there is no injury to the genital tract during the abortion • IUCD can *be inserted immediately* after postabortion
	Female sterilization	• Can be performed *concurrently* or *within 7 days* • Of abortion provided woman is eligible and fit for surgery—either minilap/laparoscopic sterilization
After medical abortion using tablet mifepristone and tablet misoprostol	Combined oral contraceptive pills—mono-/bi-/triphasic	Can be started and initiated on the third day or the 15th day of medical abortion regimen protocol. It is mandatory to rule out any contraindications for COCs
	Progestin-only contraceptive pills	Can be initiated with immediate effect
	Centchroman pills/Saheli	Can be initiated in the immediate postabortion period starting on the third day
	Injectable progesterone—injection DMPA	Can be started on the third day following medical abortion
	Condoms	Can be used by the male partner at the time of resumption of sexual activity
	IUCD	Can be inserted after the medical abortion process is completed (approximately the 15th day), after ruling out the presence of infection, or can select the first week of the next menstrual period (*Note:* on Day 15, the healthcare giver should take a detailed clinical history and do a thorough clinical examination, including a pelvic examination to ensure the absence of pelvic infection. This may also help in determining the completion of abortion; however, USG is a more reliable option to check for retained products of conception/ completion of the process of abortion)
	Female sterilization	Can be performed in the time period of the first 7 days of the immediate next menstrual cycle

Contd...

Contd...

	Family planning method	*Time of initiation after abortion*
Following second-trimester abortion		
Spontaneous abortion/surgically performed, e.g., dilatation and evacuation	Progestin-only contraceptive pills	Can be initiated with *immediate effect*
	Centchroman pills/Saheli	Can be initiated in *the immediate postabortion period starting* on the third day
	Injectable progesterone—the injection of DMPA	Can be started on the third *day after a medical abortion*
	Condoms	Can be used by the male partner whenever there is resumption of sexual activity
	IUCD	Can opt to be inserted *immediately, provided genital tract infection along with genital tract injury have been ruled out by a specially trained* provider in accordance with the PPIUCD standard protocol method
	Female sterilization	• Can be performed concurrently or in the immediate 7 days following the abortion (uncomplicated abortion), provided that the woman has made a voluntary, informed choice in advance • It is recommended to carry out the sterilization by minilap method only. (The fallopian tubes are edematous post second-trimester abortion and may result in injury during laparoscopic occlusion by rings. There are also increased chances of slippage of the rings/clips from the tubes resulting in tubectomy failures)

Note: The National Family Planning Programme offers vasectomy as male sterilization services also which can be opted for by the male partner anytime.

(COC: combined oral contraceptive; DMPA: depot medroxyprogesterone acetate; IUCD: intrauterine contraceptive device; PPIUCD: postpartum intrauterine contraceptive device; USG: ultrasound)

TABLE 2: Eligibility criteria for postabortion IUCD insertion.[1,5]

Condition	*MEC category for IUCD insertion*
In the immediate period following first-trimester abortion (either spontaneous or induced). (Provided there is no evidence or potential for developing infection)	1
In the immediate period following second-trimester abortion (either spontaneous or induced). (Provided there is no evidence or potential for developing infection and after ruling out the presence of bleeding and other contraindications)	2

(IUCD: intrauterine contraceptive device; MEC: medical eligibility criteria for contraceptive use)

TABLE 3: Clinical technique of postabortion IUCD insertion.[1,5]

Method of abortion	***Technique of insertion immediately after abortion***
After evacuation by surgical methods—S and E, D and E when uterine size is <12 weeks	The technique is similar to that of the interval IUCD insertion technique (no touch and withdrawal technique) with some modifications of the insertion steps: • Routine use of uterine sound for assessment of uterine length is not recommended, as it may cause perforation • Uterine length may be assessed right at the end of the surgical procedure, with the suction cannula being used for the evacuation, just before withdrawing out the cannula • If D and E is the method of surgical abortion being performed, the uterine length can be measured using the last curette at the time of completion of the procedure • Next, the IUCD is loaded keeping it inside the sterile package. The blue gauge present on the inserter is fixed at the length measured by the cannula • The remaining steps are the same as in the interval IUCD insertion technique (no touch and withdrawal technique)
Condition	***Clinical technique of insertion immediately after abortion***
After evacuation by surgical methods—S and E, D and E, when uterine size is >12 weeks	Similar to the technique of PPIUCD insertion with some modifications of steps: • The IUCD may be inserted using ring forceps or the sponge holder as it may be difficult in the second-trimester uterus to introduce PPIUCD insertion forceps through the internal os (The length of the uterine cavity following evacuation is much less as compared to the size of the uterus after a full-term vaginal delivery. Additionally, the cervical os may not be as patulous as is after vaginal birth. Due to these factors, difficulty may be faced while trying to introduce PPIUCD insertion forceps into the cervix. Therefore, it is advisable to do the insertion with ring forceps/sponge holder. The actual steps of insertion which need to be followed, match with those in the insertion technique of the immediate postpartum IUCD insertion)
After medical abortion using pills (mifepristone in combination with misoprostol)	Similar to the technique of insertion is of interval IUCD: • Uterine sound may be used for assessing uterine length; however, the healthcare provider needs to be very careful while introducing uterine sound into the uterine cavity • The uterine sound should be held in a way similar to holding a pen/pencil. The sound should then should be introduced very gently and carefully through the internal os. The operator needs to move it in the right direction till the resistance of the fundus is felt. This ought to be done without applying any force

(IUCD: intrauterine contraceptive device; PPIUCD: postpartum intrauterine contraceptive device)

FEMALE STERILIZATION (TUBAL LIGATION)—POSTABORTION[6,7]

- It is imperative that the woman has received counseling and made an educated choice that is based on adequate and correct information provided to her, prior to proceeding with performing a female sterilization surgery.
- The surgery should be undertaken only by healthcare providers who have been adequately trained to carry out the procedure.
- Postabortion female sterilization can be performed using the "minilap" method of tubectomy both after first and second-trimester abortions.
- Laparoscopic tubal sterilization procedure is not recommended following second-trimester abortions as there exist increased chances of injury to the fallopian tubes/uterus.

Eligibility Criteria

See **Table 4**.

TABLE 4: Eligibility criteria for postabortion female sterilization.[1,6,7]

Postabortion status	*MEC categories for female sterilization*
Uncomplicated	A
Postabortal sepsis or fever	D
Severe hemorrhage in the postabortal period	D
Intraoperative severe trauma to genital tract, cervical, or vaginal tears	D
Uterine perforation during the procedure	S
Acute hematometra	D

Note:
A: Accept—there is no reason to deny sterilization to a person with this condition
C: Caution—the procedure is normally conducted in a routine setting, but with extra precautions
D: Delay)—the procedure is delayed until the condition is evaluated and/or corrected
S: Special—the procedure should be undertaken in a setting with an experienced surgeon and staff equipment is needed to provide general anesthesia and another backup medical support

OTHER METHODS OF CONTRACEPTION

The various other methods of contraception like the combined oral contraceptive pills (OCPs), Progestin-only-pills (POPs), centchroman, injection depot medroxy-progesterone acetate (DMPA), condoms, and male sterilization if opted for, can be implemented immediately (as mentioned in earlier section), after appropriate method specific counseling and screening for eligibility.

- If the woman opts for and chooses to start OCPs, POPs, centchroman, and injection DMPA within 7 days after first or second-trimester abortion (either spontaneous or induced), there is no need for any additional backup method of contraception.
- If >7 days have elapsed after first- or second-trimester abortion (either spontaneous or induced), she can start OCPs or POPs or centchroman or injection DMPA any time if it is reasonably certain she is not pregnant. She will however need to use a backup method of contraception for the first 7 days for OCPs or injection DMPA or centchroman and for the first 2 days in case she opts for POPs.

SUMMARY AND OVERVIEW OF POSTABORTION FAMILY PLANNING METHODS[1,8,9]

See **Table 5**.

TABLE 5: Overview of postabortion family planning methods.[1,8,9]

Family planning methods	***Advantages***	***Limitations***	***Contraceptive effectiveness***
Condoms	• Only method that protects against both pregnancy and STIs and HIV • No hormonal side effects • Used as a temporary or back p method also • Can be used without needing to seek the help of a healthcare provider	• Some people may have an allergy to latex-both males and females • Requires correct and consistent use with every act of sex	• Fairly effective • *Failure rate:* Two pregnancies/100 women
Combined oral contraceptives (COCs)	• Can be provided by all health workers • Does not interfere with sexual activity • Immediate return to fertility on discontinuation	• Must be taken every day • Further supplies of the pills must be available • Not suitable for women, who are lactating and their baby is <6 months old • Not suitable for women who have certain medical illnesses • Certain medications such as rifampicin, phenytoin, and griseofulvin have drug interactions and lower the effectiveness of OCPs • Changes in menstrual bleeding, such as decreased flow of menstrual bleeding, dizziness, nausea, headaches, and breast tenderness	• Highly effective • *Failure rate:* <1 pregnancy/100 women (0.3/100), when no pills are missed
Progestin-only pills (POPs)	• Can be provided by all health workers • Does not interfere with sexual activity • Immediate return to fertility on discontinuation • Suitable even for women below 6 weeks postpartum and lactating mothers	• Less effective for women, not breastfeeding • Must be taken every day • Further pill supply must be available • Not suitable for women with certain medical illnesses • Changes in menstrual bleeding, such as decreased flow of menstrual bleeding, dizziness, nausea, headaches, and breast tenderness	• Breastfeeding women: • *Failure rate:* 1 pregnancy/100 women (0.3/100), when no pills are missed • Less effective in nonbreastfeeding women • *Failure rate:* <1 pregnancy/100 women (0.9/100), when no pills are missed

Contd...

Contd...

Family planning methods	***Advantages***	***Limitations***	***Contraceptive effectiveness***
Centchroman	• Can be used safely by lactating mothers • Does not require daily action and does not interfere with sex. Taken orally twice a week in the first 3 months and then once a week • Can be provided by nonmedical staff • Immediate return of fertility on discontinuation • No hormonal side-effects	• Prolongation of menstrual cycle • Requirement of regular supply • Cannot be provided to women with Polycystic ovarian disease, cervical hyperplasia, tuberculosis, renal disease, clinical evidence of jaundice/liver disease, and severe allergic states	• Fairly effective • *Failure rate:* 1.63 pregnancy/100 women (1.63/100)
Injection DMPA	• Does not interfere with sexual activity • Suitable for women after 6 weeks postpartum and breastfeeding	• The patient needs to return to the healthcare facility for an injection every 3 months • May cause irregular bleeding, spotting, and amenorrhea • Return of fertility after stopping Injection DMPA takes an average of 4 to 6 months. This is longer than with most other reversible methods. This means women can become pregnant on average, 7–10 months after their last injection • Reversible reductions in bone density, but users are not likely to have more fractures	• Highly effective • *Failure rate:* <1 pregnancy/100 women (0.3/100), when women take injections on

Contd...

Contd...

Family planning methods	***Advantages***	***Limitations***	***Contraceptive effectiveness***
IUCD	• Effective as soon as it is inserted • Long-term contraception, effective for 5 years (IUCD Cu 375) or 10 years (IUCD CU 380A) • Immediate return to fertility on removal • Does not require daily action and does not interfere with sex	• Increased menstrual bleeding and pain during the first few months • Trained provider needed for insertion and removal • Cannot be provided to women with current pelvic infections	• Highly effective • *Failure rate:* <1 pregnancy/100 women (0.6/100)
Female sterilization	• Permanent method • Immediately effective • No long-term side effects • No interference with sex	• Women must understand that it is a permanent method and reversal is difficult • Permanence of the method increases the importance of adequate counseling and fully informed consent • Slight possibility of surgical complications	• Highly effective • *Failure rate:* <1 pregnancy/100 women (0.5/100)
Male sterilization (vasectomy)	• Permanent method • No interference with sex • Enables man to take responsibility for preventing pregnancy	• Not immediately effective • Couple must use another FP method for at least the first 3 months. Semen analysis should be done after 3 months to confirm the absence of the sperms	• Highly effective • *Failure rate:* <1 pregnancy/100 women (0.5/100)

(DMPA: depot medroxyprogesterone acetate; IUCD: intrauterine contraceptive device)

REFERENCES

1. Ministry of Health and Family Welfare, Government of India. (2016). Operational Guidelines Post Abortion Family Planning. Annexure A. [online] Available from http://www.nrhmtn.gov.in/guideline/PostAboFPGlines.pdf. [Last accessed January, 2023].
2. World Health Organization. Unsafe Abortion: Global and Regional Estimates of the Incidence of Unsafe Abortion and Associated Mortality in 2008, 6th edition. Geneva: World Health Organization; 2011.
3. Mesce D. In: Carnevale E (Ed). Unsafe Abortion: Facts and Figures. Washington DC: Population Reference Bureau; 2005.
4. World Health Organization. Trends in Maternal mortality: 1990 to 2013, Estimates by WHO, UNICEF, UNFPA, The World Bank and the United Nations Population Division. Geneva: World Health Organization; 2014.
5. Nguyen Thi Nhu Ngoc. Immediate post-abortion insertion of intrauterine devices: RHL commentary. Geneva: The WHO Reproductive Health Library; 2005.
6. Ministry of Health & Family Welfare; Government of India. (2014). Reference Manual for Female Sterilization. [online] Available from https://cghealth.nic.in/dhs/NEW%20OFFERINGS-FP%20GUIDELINES/Ref%20Manual%20for%20Female%20Sterilization%202014.pdf [Last accessed January, 2023].
7. Ministry of Health & Family Welfare; Government of India. (2014). Standards and Quality Assurance in Sterilization Services. [online] Available from https://nhm.gov.in/images/pdf/programmes/family-planing/guidelines/Standards_and_Quality_Assurance.pdf [Last accessed January, 2023].
8. Maternal Health Division, MOHFW, Govt. of India. (2018). Provider's Manual on Comprehensive Abortion Care. [online] Available from https://nhm.gov.in/New_Updates_2018/NHM_Components/RMNCHA/MH/Guidelines/CAC_Training_and_Service_Delivery_Guideline.pdf [Last accessed January, 2023].
9. IPAS. In: Kapp N (Ed). Clinical Updates in Reproductive Health. Chapel Hill, NC: Ipas; 2021.

CHAPTER 22

Contraception after Ectopic Pregnancy

Ashish Kale, Ashwini Kale

INTRODUCTION AND BACKGROUND

The incidence of ectopic pregnancy is around 1.5–2%.[1]

It is important to advise a patient to use some form of contraception, who has just completed treatment of "ectopic" pregnancy, as history of ectopic pregnancy is risk factor for repeat ectopic pregnancy.[2]

COUNSELING FOR CONTRACEPTION AFTER ECTOPIC PREGNANCY

Women are willing to opt for any contraception after treatment completion of ectopic pregnancy due to following reasons: (a) Women is not pregnant; (b) Her motivation is at the highest level; and (c) She is already coming to hospital.

Women who have just completed treatment of ectopic pregnancy and wish to choose contraception, be given various options of contraception, while ensuring that they do not come under any kind of pressure to choose particular contraceptive method.

As women have gone through trauma of ectopic pregnancy, they are ready to choose any form of contraception till they decide future family planning.

It is ideal to initiate some method of contraception immediately after treatment completion of ectopic pregnancy. This is especially more important in the cases in which ectopic pregnancy has been treated with injection "methotrexate". Patient should compulsorily use some method of contraception during and after treatment for minimum period of 3 months to avoid teratogenic effects of injection methotrexate.

Till the women decide to use type of contraception, at least some form of bridging method should be used to avoid pregnancy.

VARIOUS TYPES OF CONTRACEPTIVE METHODS

Combine Hormonal Contraceptive Pills

After counseling of the patients, combine hormonal contraceptive pills may be started when the treatment of the ectopic pregnancy gets completed.

Progesterone Only Pills

- After counseling of the patients, progesterone only pills (POPs) may be started when the treatment of the ectopic pregnancy gets completed.
- Intramuscular depot medroxyprogesterone acetate (DMPA) or progesterone only implant, if available, is a good option.

Intrauterine Devices

Intrauterine copper devices or levonorgestrel intrauterine releasing system (LNG-IUS) may be prescribed to patients of ectopic pregnancy excluding the cases of sepsis.

Barrier Methods

- After counseling of the patient, any male or female barrier method may be advised after treatment of ectopic pregnancy get completed. As failure rate of condoms is very high, they should be preferred as last option **(Table 1)**.
- Barrier method or abstinence should be used if combine hormonal contraceptive pills, POPs, progesterone only implant or injection, and LNG-IUS are started 5 days after completion of treatment of ectopic pregnancy.

TABLE 1: Failure rate of various contraceptive methods.[3]

Methods	*Typical use (%)*	*Perfect use (%)*
No use	85	85
Fertility awareness based methods	24	0.4–5
Female diaphragm	12	6
Male condom	18	2
Combined hormonal contraception	9	0.3
Progesterone only pills	9	0.3
Injection progesterone only	6	0.2
Copper intrauterine device	0.8	0.6
Levonorgestrel releasing intrauterine system	0.2	0.2
Progesterone only implant	0.05	0.05
Female sterilization	0.5	0.5
Vasectomy	0.15	0.1

Fertility Awareness Methods

Have very high failure rate and patient should be counseled thoroughly regarding it.

Female Sterilization

- It is a good option especially for the patient who are undergoing surgery for removal of ectopic pregnancy.
- Also, it can also be offered to patient postmedical treatment of ectopic pregnancy.

EMERGENCY CONTRACEPTION AFTER ECTOPIC PREGNANCY

It is advisable to opt for emergency contraception if there is unprotected sexual intercourse 5 days after taking injection methotrexate or surgical treatment of ectopic pregnancy.

REFERENCES

1. Barnhart KT. Clinical practice. Ectopic pregnancy. N Engl J Med. 2009;361:379-87.
2. Juneau C, Bates GW. Reproductive outcomes after medical and surgical management of ectopic pregnancy. Clin Obstet Gynecol. 2012;55:455-60.
3. The Faculty of Sexual and Reproductive Healthcare. (2020). FSRH Clinical Guideline Contraception After Pregnancy (January 2017, amended October 2020). [online] Available from: https://www.fsrh.org/standards-and-guidance/documents/contraception-after-pregnancy-guideline-january-2017/ [Last accessed November, 2022].

CHAPTER 23

Good Clinical Practice Recommendations on Combined Hormonal Contraceptives: Counseling and Use in Clinical Practice

Ashwini Kale, Ashish Kale

INTRODUCTION

According to the third National Family Health Survey (NFHS-3), which was conducted in 2005–2006 in India, 98% of women and 99% of men aged 15–49 years were aware of one or more methods of contraception.[1] In contrast, the Demographic Health Survey Data for India (2005–2006) revealed that 52% of illiterate women do not use any method of contraception.[2] Given that such women are mainly from low-income households and have limited access to healthcare services, they comprise a particularly vulnerable section of the community.

Contraceptive use has been increasing in India over the last few decades. Oral contraceptives are being used by more than 100 million women worldwide, which vary generally by country, age, education, and marital status.[3] The most common methods of hormonal contraception include the combined hormonal contraceptive (CHC) pill and the mini-pill.[4] Currently, many newer brands of CHCs use lower estrogen doses that have increased safety with equal efficacy.[5]

AIM AND PURPOSE

Combined hormonal contraceptives belong to a group of hormonal contraceptives, which are one of the most effective methods of preventing pregnancy. The current recommendations focus on the use of CHCs in routine clinical scenario and the importance of structured counseling to patients. The objectives are as follows:

- To enhance the awareness on contraception
- To update physicians on CHC effectiveness and safety
- To encourage acceptance of CHC in Indian women
- To dispel the myths/misconceptions around CHC
- To update additional health benefits of CHC
- To reassure safe use of CHC by providing comprehensive information to users.

GOOD CLINICAL PRACTICE RECOMMENDATIONS METHODOLOGY

The good clinical practice recommendations (GCPR) methodology for developing the guidelines is as follows:

- The clinical evidence for the guidelines were taken from global studies.
- The guidelines were developed and reviewed by the expert committee of the Federation of Obstetric and Gynecological Societies of India (FOGSI).
- The guidelines were eventually finalized to be used by the healthcare providers.

ROLE OF COMBINED HORMONAL CONTRACEPTIVES

Despite an overall decline in maternal mortality rate from 212 (in 2007–2009) to 178 in 2012, India still lags behind the target of 103 deaths per live births to be achieved by 2015 under the United Nations-mandated Millennium Development Goals (MDG).

Combined hormonal contraceptives certainly have a great impact on reducing unwanted pregnancies and associated sociomedical morbidity.[6] They are considered as an extremely effective method of contraception and also have health benefits beyond pregnancy prevention. CHCs can provide relief from symptoms associated with menstruation including heavy menstrual bleeding (HMB), dysmenorrhea, and irregular bleeding, thus reducing the risk of iron deficiency anemia by about 50%. CHCs also offer several important health benefits unrelated to birth control, which include reduced risk of benign ovarian disease, ovarian and endometrial cancer, and benign breast disease.[7]

PATIENT'S EXPECTATIONS FROM MODERN-DAY CONTRACEPTIVE

Contraceptive Efficacy

When used correctly, CHCs are an effective method of contraception as evident by their low Pearl Index. They also confer health benefits beyond pregnancy prevention.

Safety with Few Side Effects

Combined hormonal contraceptives offer an effective, convenient, tolerable, and well-accepted method of hormonal contraception.

Relief from Menstrual Symptoms

Combined hormonal contraceptives reduce the risk of iron deficiency anemia by 50% and provide almost immediate relief from troublesome symptoms associated with menstruation, including heavy periods, dysmenorrhea, premenstrual dysphoric disorder (PMDD), and irregular bleeding.

Return to Fertility

Irrespective of duration of use of CHC, complete return to fertility usually occurs immediately after stopping CHC use.[8]

COMBINED HORMONAL CONTRACEPTIVES OPTIONS AVAILABLE IN INDIA

Combined Oral Contraceptive Pills

Combined oral contraceptives (COCs) consist of a combination of estrogen and progestin.

Estrogen: The past two decades have witnessed a trend toward lowering the ethinyl estradiol (EE) dosing. Formulations are available with EE dosing, ranging from 50 (high dose) to 20 µg (ultralow dose) but mostly are of 30–35 µg (low dose).

Progestins: They are classified based on their sequence of development as follows[9] (*Note*: The definitions are not universally accepted.):

- *First generation:* Estranes and pregnanes
  - Estranes derived from 19-nortestosterone, e.g., norethisterone acetate and lynestrenol
  - Estranes derived from 17-hydroxyprogesterone, e.g., medroxyprogesterone acetate, cyproterone acetate, and chlormadinone acetate
- *Second generation:* Gonanes, e.g., levonorgestrel (LNG) or norgestrel
- *Third generation:* Gonanes, e.g., gestodene, desogestrel, and norgestimate
- *Fourth generation:*
  - 19-norpregnanes, e.g., nestorone, nomegestrol acetate, and trimegestone

- Estranes (non-ethinylated), e.g., dienogest
- Spironolactone derivative, e.g., drospirenone (DRSP).

Pharmacology of Combined Oral Contraceptives

Ethinyl estradiol is metabolized at several different sites. First, it is sulfated in the intestinal wall, then it is hydroxylated in the liver through the cytochrome P450 pathway, after which it is conjugated with glucuronides and passed into the enterohepatic circulation. Drug interactions may occur via alterations in absorption, serum protein binding, and receptor binding or hepatic metabolism **(Table 1)**.

Combined Oral Contraceptive Preparations

Monophasic: Each pill contains fixed amount of estrogen and progestin. They come in various regimens and administrations, such as 21/7, 24/4, or 84/7 regimens.

Biphasic: In biphasic preparation, the estrogen component remains fixed, while the amount of progestin increases in the second half of the cycle.

Triphasic: The amount of estrogen dose in triphasic preparation may be fixed or variable, while the amount of progestin increases in three equal phases.

Biphasic and triphasic preparations were developed to reduce the total steroid content of COCs.[11]

Quadriphasic: Quadriphasic preparations have been developed to reduce the side effects of oral contraceptives and are considered more physiological since they mimic the natural cycle.[12,13] Currently, there is one quadriphasic preparation available and it contains estradiol valerate 3 mg on days 1 and 2; dienogest 2 mg and estradiol valerate 2 mg on days 3–7; dienogest 3 mg and estradiol valerate 2 mg on days 8–24; estradiol valerate 1 mg on days 25 and 26; and placebo on days 27 and 28; however, it is not currently available in India.

Continuous or Extended Cycle: Continuous or extended cycle preparation involves the intake of active pills (generally 84/7 regimen), whereby the dose of estrogen increases at three distinct

TABLE 1: Major drug interactions with combined oral contraceptives (COCs).[10]

Medications whose action may cause contraception failure	***Medications which may increase COC activity***	***Medications whose clearance can be decreased by COCs***
Carbamazepine	Acetaminophen	Amitriptyline
Griseofulvin	Erythromycin	Caffeine
Oxcarbazepine	Fluoxetine	Cyclosporine
Phenobarbital	Fluconazole	Diazepam
Phenytoin	Fluvoxamine	Imipramine
Primidone	Grapefruit juice	Phenytoin
Rifampin	Nefazodone	Selegiline
Ritonavir	Vitamin C	Theophylline
St John's Wort		
Topiramate		

points over the first 84 days and the amount of progestin remains constant; this is followed by 7 days of inactive or low-dose estrogen pills. This has shown to have advantages such as decreased incidence of pelvic pain, headaches, bloating/swelling, breast tenderness, improvement in symptoms of endometriosis, and polycystic ovary syndrome.[14-16]

Regimens of Administration

21/7 Regimen: The 21/7 regimen contains the same amount and combination of estrogen and progestin in each of the 21 active pills followed by 7 days of hormone-free interval.

24/4 Regimen: The 24/4 regimen consists of 24 active pills and 4 placebo or folate tablets, which are distinguished by a different color.

26/2 Regimen: In the 26/2 regimen, hormones of varying doses are taken every day for 26 days, while the last two pills contain no active substances.

Extended day Regimen: The 84 + 7 day regimen contains 84 days of estrogen and progestin, followed by 7 days of either placebo or very low-dose estrogen (10 μg/day). These products are designed for the occurrence of four withdrawal bleeds per year.[17]

Continuous Hormone Regimen: Continuous hormone regimen contains EE 20 μg and LNG 90 μg. This product is packaged like a 28-day regimen, but each pill pack contains 28 days of active hormones, taken continuously with no hormone-free interval to induce scheduled withdrawal bleeding.[18-20]

Initiation of Combined Oral Contraceptive

"Sunday start" method: Conventionally, the COC is started during the first 5 days of the menstrual cycle or on the first Sunday after menses begin. If the COC is started within the first 5 days of the menstrual cycle, a backup method of contraception is not necessary for prevention of pregnancy, provided that no pills have been missed.[10]

"Quick start" method: Initiation on any day of the cycle is referred to as the "quick start" method. This eliminates the delay between receiving a prescription and starting the new contraceptive method which may improve adherence. "Quick start" method significantly improves the continuation rate for COCs, reduces the likelihood of a potential unplanned pregnancy, and results in better adherence.[21,22] However, one drawback with this method would be an inadvertent use of COC pill during an undetected pregnancy.[22]

Postabortion use/after miscarriage: After an abortion before 12 weeks of gestation, oral contraceptives should be started immediately to inhibit the ovulation which may occur 2 weeks after the abortion. If the abortion is of more than 12 weeks of gestation, oral contraceptives should be started 1 week after the termination because of the uncertainty of the time of ovulation with regard to the first menstruation.[23]

Postpartum use: If the woman has just delivered and is not breastfeeding, the COC pill can be started on day 21 after the birth. If the pill is started later than 21 days after the birth, an additional contraception is required for the next 7 days. If the female is breastfeeding and the baby is less than 6 months old, taking the COC pill can reduce the flow of milk. It is recommended to use an alternate method of contraception until breastfeeding is discontinued.

Vaginal Rings

Pharmacology

The vaginal ring is a nonbiodegradable, flexible, soft, copolymer ring that is placed inside the vagina. It is about 4 mm thick and 54 mm in diameter. When inserted, vaginal rings release, on an average, 120 µg/day of etonogestrel and 15 µg/day of EE over a 3-week period of use.[24] This allows for lower doses, greater bioavailability, and good cycle control.

Current prototypes in development include rings releasing progesterone receptor modulators, which would provide estrogen-free contraception, as well as combined rings releasing estradiol, having a better safety profile.

Regimen

The ring is inserted into the vagina and used continuously for 3 weeks. It is removed for a 1-week break period, during which a withdrawal bleed usually occurs. A new ring is inserted after 1 week.

Initiation and Use of Ring

The ring needs to be inserted on day 1 of menstrual bleeding. However if it is started on days 2–5, then an additional method of contraception should be followed for 7 days.

Postabortion use/after miscarriage: The ring can be inserted within the first 5 days following complete first trimester abortion or miscarriage, in which case no additional method of contraception is required.

Postpartum use: If the woman has just delivered and is not breastfeeding, the ring should be used no sooner than 4 weeks. However, women who are breastfeeding should be advised not to use the ring and to use other forms of contraception until the child is weaned or after 6 months from delivery.

Inadvertent removal/expulsion: If the ring is accidentally expelled, it has to be rinsed with lukewarm water and reinserted as soon as possible, but at the latest within 3 hours.

Insertion and Removal of the Ring

To insert the vaginal ring, it should be squeezed between the thumb and index finger and gently inserted toward the posterior fornix, allowing it to take a comfortable position in the vagina.

The vaginal ring is removed by hooking it with the index finger and gently pulling it out.

Injectables

Pharmacology

Though not available in India yet, a monthly injectable contraceptive comprising 5 mg estradiol cypionate and 25 mg medroxyprogesterone acetate was approved by the United States Food and Drug Administration (USFDA) in October, 2000.[10] Estradiol cypionate gave significantly lower peak levels of estradiol and estrone than estradiol enanthate and valerate. Also, as it is administered by injection, the first-pass metabolism by the liver is avoided, thereby minimizing estradiol's effect on the liver.

Regimen

The contraceptive injection is usually given intramuscularly with no more than a month's gap between injections. The vaginal bleeding with this method is due to estrogen withdrawal and usually occurs 3 weeks (day 22) after the injection.[25]

Initiation and Use of Injectables

The contraceptive injection (0.5 mL) is administered intramuscularly into the deltoid, gluteus maximus, or anterior thigh.

First injection:

- Within the first 5 days of the onset of a normal menstrual period
- Within 5 days of a complete first trimester abortion

- No earlier than 4 weeks of postpartum if not breastfeeding
- No earlier than 6 weeks of postpartum if breastfeeding

Second and subsequent injections: Subsequent injections every month should be administered within 28–30 days after the previous injection and should not exceed 33 days.

If the patient has not adhered to the prescribed schedule (>33 days since last injection), pregnancy should be considered and she should not receive another injection until pregnancy is ruled out.

NONCONTRACEPTIVE BENEFITS OF COMBINED HORMONAL CONTRACEPTIVE

The noncontraceptive benefits of CHCs are not only an added advantage to women who use this method but also have an important public health benefit. Currently, CHCs are increasingly prescribed for noncontraceptive indications.

Noncontraceptive Indications

Acne

Combined oral contraceptives provide considerable improvement in signs of hyperandrogenism which include acne and hirsutism.[26] COCs with newer progestins such as DRSP having antiandrogenic activity are additionally indicated in mild-to-moderate acne.

Premenstrual Dysphoric Disorder

The 24/4 regimen containing a newer progestin DRSP is additionally indicated for relief from physical and emotional symptoms of PMDD with improvements in health-related quality of life.[26] Using extended cycle or continuous CHC regimens to suppress menstruation and stabilize hormone levels also seems to be effective.

Noncontraceptive Benefits

Menstrual Irregularities and Dysmenorrhea

Combined hormonal contraceptives are often used as therapeutic drugs for women with HMB and dysmenorrhea. COCs are generally used to manage heavy and intermenstrual bleeding by restoring synchrony to the endometrium. COCs in conjunction with nonsteroidal anti-inflammatory medications have also been postulated as first-line treatment for dysmenorrhea.[27]

Anemia

Combined oral contraceptives decrease menstrual blood loss and regulate menstrual bleeding, thus reducing the likelihood of iron-deficiency anemia by almost 50%. This benefits both current and past users of COCs.[27]

Endometriosis

Combined oral contraceptives can be considered as an alternative treatment for the painful symptoms of endometriosis. COCs have an advantage over danazol or other gonadotropin hormone-releasing hormone (GnRH) agonists in having a better long-term tolerability profile.[27]

Bone Mineral Density

Combined oral contraceptives have been reported to have nil or even beneficial effects on bone mineral density (BMD). Their use in later reproductive years is associated with increased BMD and longer duration of use with greater BMD.[26]

Perimenopausal Hormonal Replacement Therapy

For women with premature (age <40 years) or early (<45 years) menopause, hormone replacement therapy (HRT) is recommended until the age of 51 years for the treatment of vasomotor symptoms and bone preservation.[28] A woman who is under 50 years and free of all risk factors for venous and arterial thrombosis can use a low-dose COC to provide relief from menopausal symptoms and for increasing BMD.

Endometrial/Colorectal/Ovarian Cancer

Combined oral contraceptives confer a 50% risk reduction from endometrial cancer with longer duration of use associated with greater risk reductions and lasts up to 20 years.

Combined oral contraceptives have also been shown to reduce the risk of colorectal cancer by 18% and ovarian cancer by approximately 20% for every 5 years of use. This protective effect also extends to low-dose pills.[26]

ROLE OF COUNSELING

Structured contraception counseling using standardized protocol and aids have shown to significantly increase the selection of modern contraceptive methods.[29] Adequate counseling prior to initiation of any CHCs helps in improving compliance (regular use) and adherence (continuation). Counseling is a key element in providing quality care and is also an important part of both initiation and follow-up visits. Women should be given adequate information with respect to effectiveness of contraception, correct use, common side effects, and health risks and benefits, along with dispelling any myths in order to help make an informed and voluntary choice.

Counseling for Combined Oral Contraceptives

Patient Assessment

- A thorough clinical history must be taken, which comprises current and previous medical conditions and menstrual and medication history.
- Specifically enquire about risk factors such as smoking, obesity, hypertension, thrombophilia, previous venous thromboembolism (VTE), and hyperlipidemia.
- The patients' preference and concerns about the COCs must be addressed.
- Blood pressure, body weight, and preferably body mass index (BMI) should be recorded.
- COCs should be used in caution with patients who are on liver enzyme inducers, e.g., antiepileptic and antitubercular drugs.

Initiating Combined Oral Contraceptive Regimen

First-time users should be prescribed a low-dose COC containing no more than 35 μg EE.[30] Before starting a contraceptive pill, it is important to ensure that the woman fulfils the criteria of eligibility for use.

There are various regimens of COCs available and she should be informed about them. She should also be counseled regarding their proper use as well as management of missed pills.

"Missed pill"

Contraceptive pills can be started any time in the menstrual cycle if the woman is sure that she is not pregnant. It is very important to counsel and instruct woman in case of missed/delayed pills.

Recommended actions after late or missed Combined oral contraceptives (monophasic)[17]
Missed 1 pill but less than 24 hours late (regardless of pill week): Take a tablet as soon as possible and continue regimen as prescribed (this measure means that in some cases, two pills will be taken on one day).

Missed ≥1 pill in first week of the pill packet: Take the last missed pill as soon as possible and continue regimen as prescribed (this measure means that in some cases, two pills will be taken on one day); additional contraception for 7 days; consider emergency contraception (if unprotected sex has occurred in the last 5 days).

Missed <3 pills (in the 2nd or 3rd week of pill packet): Take the last missed pill as soon as possible and continue regimen as prescribed (this measure means that in some cases, two pills will be taken on one day); omit the pill-free interval before beginning the next pill packet.

Missed ≥3 pills (in the 2nd or 3rd week of pill packet): Take the last missed pill as soon as possible and continue regimen as prescribed (this measure means that in some cases, two pills will be taken on one day); omit the pill-free interval before beginning the next pill packet; additional contraception for 7 days; consider emergency contraception (where several pills have been missed or there has been a greater than 7-day period with no pills taken).

Noncontraceptive Benefits

Patients should be counseled that apart from providing excellent contraception, COCs also help in the reduction of HMB and dysmenorrhea, reduction in the risk of ovarian, endometrial, and colorectal cancer, and improvement in acne vulgaris.[31,32]

Also, pills with newer progestins such as DRSP having antimineralocorticoid activity lead to minimal or no "pill-related" weight gain.

Side Effects

Side effects are generally experienced during the first 3 months with the most common being abnormal menstrual bleeding, followed by nausea, weight gain, mood changes, breast tenderness, and headache. Reassurance and adequate counseling about expected common side effects can help to prevent discontinuation and enhance compliance.

Combined Oral Contraceptives and Risk of Cancer

Combined oral contraceptive reduces the risks of ovarian, endometrial, and colorectal cancer. This reduced risk has also been noted in women who have a pathogenic mutation in the *BRCA1* or *BRCA2* gene.

Research is being carried out to assess the role of COCs and the risk of cervical cancer as virtually all cervical cancers are caused by persistent infection with high-risk or oncogenic types of human papillomavirus (HPV), and the association of cervical cancer with oral contraceptive use is likely to be indirect.[33] As the risk of these events is very small, women should be carefully counseled regarding the same.

Counseling for Vaginal Rings

Patient Assessment

Patient assessment is similar to COCs mentioned earlier.

Initiating Vaginal Rings

Though it is advisable to get the vaginal ring inserted by a healthcare professional, it is easy to insert and can be placed in the vagina by the woman herself. After 3 weeks, the ring is removed and a new ring inserted with a gap of no more than 7 days.

If there is a problem with intercourse, the ring can be removed for up to 3 hours without loss of efficacy.

The ring can be inadvertently expelled from the vagina during removal of a tampon or bowel and bladder emptying, especially with straining and constipation. If the ring is out for more than 3 hours in the first or second week of usage, it can be rinsed with lukewarm water and reinserted. Additional contraception should be used for the next 7 days.

Noncontraceptive Benefits

Noncontraceptive benefits are similar to COCs mentioned earlier.

Side Effects

Side effects commonly experienced with ring are irregular uterine bleeding, vaginitis, nausea, weight gain, mood changes, breast tenderness, and headache. Reassurance and adequate counseling about expected common side effects can help to prevent discontinuation and enhance compliance.[10]

Counseling for Injectables

Patient Assessment

Patient assessment is similar to COCs mentioned earlier.

Initiating Injectables

Though not yet available in India, they are administered by intramuscular injection into the deltoid, gluteus maximus, or anterior thigh. Patient should be counseled to adhere with the administration routine.

Side Effects

Side effects include unscheduled vaginal bleeding, weight gain, headaches, mood swings, breast tenderness, and nausea.

SAFETY CONCERNS WITH COMBINED HORMONAL CONTRACEPTIVES

Venous Thromboembolism

Uses of CHCs are generally considered as a serious risk factor for VTE (deep vein thrombosis and pulmonary embolism).

The incidence of venous thromboembolic disease in healthy women of reproductive age is very low, at around 4–5/10,000 women per year.[34] COC use alters clotting factors and fibrinolysis via its effect on liver metabolism and can lead to a reversible activated protein C resistance (APCR). These effects contribute to an increased VTE risk with COC use of 9–10/10,000 woman years, a risk which is proportionate to the estradiol dose and highest at the beginning of treatment. By comparison, this risk during pregnancy is around 29/10,000 and in the postpartum period, around 300–400/10,000 woman years.[17]

Women should be advised that although the risk of VTE with CHC is slightly higher than nonuser, the risk is still considerably lower than the risk of VTE in pregnancy and postpartum.

Myocardial Infarction

The increased risk of myocardial infarction (MI) in young women taking COCs is marginal. Additional risk factors such as age, hypertension, smoking, diabetes, hyperlipidemia, and high BMI must also be taken into account. In women taking COCs with EE dose of 50 μg or higher, MI risk increases threefold. However, the risk of MI seen with doses <50 μg of EE is insignificant, irrespective of age. Nonsmokers at any age with no specific risk factors can be advised that they have no increased risk of MI with CHC use.

For women ≥35 years and who smoke ≥15 cigarettes per day, CHCs are not indicated and an alternative contraceptive method should be recommended.[10] Also, hypertensive patients with systolic pressure of 160 mm Hg or over and diastolic pressures of 100 mm Hg or over, COC should not be used and an alternative contraceptive method should be recommended.[17]

Stroke

Women should be counseled regarding a very small risk of ischemic stroke with CHC use. Patients with history of stroke should not be prescribed high doses of COCs. Other risk factors such as smoking, hypertension, diabetes mellitus, and MI should also be considered as they have a compounding effect, thus leading to higher chances of complications.

Breast Cancer

Numerous recent studies have concluded that the COC has either no influence or a very small influence on breast cancer.[17] History of benign breast disease or a family history of breast cancer should not be regarded as contraindication to CHC use. Women aged over 40 years should be advised that any increase in risk of breast cancer associated with CHC use is likely to be small and is in addition to their own background risk which increases with age. Also, any increase in the risk of breast cancer is reduced to no additional risk 10 years after stopping the CHC.[35]

Cervical Cancer

Human papillomavirus is the main etiology for cervical cancer. Women using oral contraceptives are more likely to be exposed to HPV than are those using barrier methods or not having sexual intercourse and should be counseled regarding the risks. Cervical screening is not 100% accurate but regular attendance reduces a woman's chance of developing cervical cancer by between 80% and 90%. Long-term use (≥5 years) of COCs is associated with a small increased risk of cervical cancer. However, the overall risk of cervical cancer is very low whether hormonal contraception is used or not and the level of risk in COC users decreases to the risk seen in nonusers within 10 years of stopping use.[36]

ELIGIBILITY CRITERIA FOR COMBINED HORMONAL CONTRACEPTION IN SPECIAL SITUATIONS[37] (TABLE 2)

Recommendations

- Method can be used without restriction
- Advantages of method generally outweigh risks
- Method not usually recommended unless other more appropriate methods are not available or not acceptable
- Method not to be used.

CONCLUSION

This GCPR regarding the CHC usage in Indian women is focused on the unmet need for the CHCs, their usage (contraceptive as well as noncontraceptive), side effects, and the importance of structured counseling to patients. We have also tried to stress the relevant safety concerns with CHCs, including contraception in special situations and patient counseling tips for a better prescribing pattern along with customizing its usage as per the patient needs.

TABLE 2: Combined hormonal contraceptive methods.

Condition	Qualifier for condition	*Combined hormonal contraceptive methods*		
		COC	*Vaginal rings*	*Combined injectables*
Lactation	<6 weeks postpartum	4	4	4
	≥6 weeks to <6 months postpartum (primarily breastfeeding)	3	3	3
	≥6 months postpartum	2	2	2
Hypertension	During prior pregnancy, now resolved	2	2	2
	Well controlled	3	3	3
	Systolic BP 140–159 mm Hg or diastolic BP 90–99 mm Hg	3	3	3
	Systolic BP ≥160 mm Hg or diastolic BP ≥100 mm Hg	4	4	4
	With vascular disease	4	4	4
Valvular heart disease	Uncomplicated	2	2	2
	Complicated	4	4	4
Ischemic heart disease	Past or current	4	4	4
Smoking	Age <35 years	2	2	2
	Age ≥35 years, <15 cigarettes per day	3	3	2
	Age ≥35 years, ≥15 cigarettes per day	4	4	3
Migraine	Without aura, age <35 years	2/3	2/3	2/3
	Without aura, age ≥35 years	3/4	3/4	3/4
	With aura, at any age	4	4	4
Thyroid disease	Simple goiter, hyperthyroidism, and hypothyroidism	1	1	1
Diabetes mellitus	History of gestational disease	1	1	1
	Without vascular disease	2	2	2
	With end-organ damage or >20 years' duration	3/4	3/4	3/4
Liver disease	Cirrhosis, mild	1	1	1
	Cirrhosis, severe	4	4	3
	Tumors, benign	2	2	2
	Tumors, malignant	4	4	4
	Viral hepatitis, carrier	1	1	1
	Viral hepatitis, active	2	2	2

Contd...

Contd...

Condition	**Qualifier for condition**	***Combined hormonal contraceptive methods***		
		COC	***Vaginal rings***	***Combined injectables***
Gallbladder disease	Asymptomatic gallstones	2	2	2
	Symptomatic gallstones, without cholecystectomy	3	3	2
	Gallstones treated with cholecystectomy	2	2	2
	Pregnancy-related cholestasis in past	2	2	2
	Hormone-related cholestasis in past	3	3	2
Antimicrobial therapy	Broad-spectrum antibiotics	1	1	1
	Antifungals	1	1	1
	Antiparasitics	1	1	1
	Rifampicin or rifabutin therapy	3	3	3
Antiretroviral therapy	NRTIs	1	1	1
	NNRTIs	2	2	2
	Ritonavir-boosted protease inhibitors	3	3	3

(BP: blood pressure; COC: combined oral contraceptive; NNRTIs: non-nucleoside reverse transcriptase inhibitors; NRTIs: nucleoside reverse transcriptase inhibitors)

REFERENCES

1. International Institute for Population Sciences. (2007). National Family Health Survey (NFHS-3) 2005-06, volume 1. [online] Available from: https://dhsprogram.com/pubs/pdf/frind3/frind3-vol1andvol2.pdf [Last accessed January, 2024].
2. Dixit P. Linkages between Unintended Births and Contraceptive Discontinuations in India. Sci Rep. 2012;1:554.
3. Shafiq M, Sheikh SA, Hassan SH. Combined oral contraceptive pills improve lung function variables. Pak J Physiol. 2012;8(1):1-5.
4. Spencer AL, Bonnema R, McNamara MC. Helping women choose appropriate hormonal contraception: update on risks, benefits, and indications. Am J Med. 2009; 122:497-506.
5. Sylvia L, Yeager BF. Update on Oral Contraceptive Pills. Am Fam Physician. 1999; 60:2073-84.
6. Baird AS, Porter CC. Teenage pregnancy: strategies for prevention. Obstet Gynaecol Reprod Med. 2011;21(6):151-7.
7. Mishell DR Jr. Noncontraceptive health benefits of oral steroidal contraceptives. Am J Obstet Gynecol. 1982;142(6 Pt 2): 809-16.
8. Department of Reproductive Health and Research Family and Community Health: World Health Organization. Selected practice recommendations for contraceptive use, 2nd edition. Geneva: World Health Organization; 2004.
9. Nath A, Sitruk-Ware R. Different cardiovascular effects of progestins according to structure and activity. Climacteric. 2009; 12(Suppl 1):96-101.
10. Black A, Francoeur D, Rowe T, Collins J, Miller D, Brown T, et al. SOGC Clinical Practice Guidelines: Canadian Contraception Consensus. J Obstet Gynaecol Can. 2004;26(3):219-96.

11. Upton GC. The phasic approach to oral contraception: the triphasic concept and its application. Int J Fertil. 1983;28:121-40.
12. Beers MH, Fletcher AJ (Eds). The Merck Manual of Medical Information, 2nd home edition. Whitehouse Station, NJ: Merck; 2003.
13. Estradiol + dienogest. Oral contraception: estradiol does not provide a therapeutic advantage. Prescrire Int. 2010;19(106):65-7.
14. Sulak P, Kuehl T, Ortiz M, Shull B. Acceptance of altering the standard 21-day/7-day oral contraceptive regimen to delay menses and reduce hormonal withdraw symptoms. Am J Obstet Gynecol. 2002;186:1142-9.
15. Vercellini P, De Giorgi O, Mosconi P, Stellato G, Vicentini S, Crosignani PG. Cyproterone acetate versus a continuous monophasic oral contraceptive in the treatment of recurrent pelvic pain after conservative surgery for symptomatic endometriosis. Fertil Steril. 2002;77(1):52-61.
16. Falsetti L, Galbignani E. Long-term treatment with the combination ethinyl estradiol and cyproterone acetate in polycystic ovary syndrome. Contraception. 1990;42(6): 611-9.
17. Wiegratz I, Thaler CJ. Hormonal contraception—what kind, when, and for whom? Dtsch Arztebl Int. 2011;108(28-29): 495-505.
18. Miller L, Hughes JP. Continuous combination oral contraceptive pills to eliminate withdrawal bleeding: a randomized trial. Obstet Gynecol. 2003;101:653-61.
19. Archer DF, Jensen JT, Johnson JV, Borisute H, Grub GS, Constantine GD. Evaluation of a continuous regimen of levonorgestrel/ethinyl estradiol: phase 3 study results. Contraception. 2006;74:439-45.
20. Edelman AB, Gallo MF, Jensen JT, Nichols MD, Schulz KF, Grimes DA. Continuous or extended cycle versus cyclic use of combined oral contraceptives for contraception. Cochrane Database Syst Rev. 2005;3: CD004695.
21. Lara-Torre E, Schroeder B. Adolescent compliance and side effects with quick start initiation of oral contraceptive pills. Contraception. 2002;66:81-5.
22. Lopez LM, Newmann SJ, Grimes DA, Nanda K, Schulz KF. Immediate start of hormonal contraceptives for contraception. Cochrane Database Syst Rev. 2008;(2):CD006260.
23. When to start the pill after abortion. Fam Plann Inf Serv. 1978;1(1):17.
24. Timmer CJ, Mulders TM. Pharmacokinetics of etonogestrel and ethinyl estradiol released from a combined contraceptive vaginal ring. Clin Pharmacokinet. 2000;39(3):233-42.
25. Garceau RJ, Wajszczuk CJ, Kaunitz AM. Bleeding patterns of women using Lunelle monthly contraceptive injections (medroxyprogesterone acetate and estradiol cypionate injectable suspension) compared with those of women using Ortho-Novum 7/7/7 (norethindrone/ethinyl estradiol triphasic) or other oral contraceptives. Contraception. 2002;62(6):289-95.
26. Armstrong C. ACOG Guidelines on Non-contraceptive Uses of Hormonal Contraceptives. Am Fam Physician. 2010; 82(3):288-95.
27. Dayal M, Barnhart KT. Non-contraceptive Benefits and Therapeutic Uses of the Oral Contraceptive Pill. Semin Reprod Med. 2001;19(4):295-303.
28. Hickey M, Elliott J, Davison SL. Hormone replacement therapy. BMJ. 2012;344:e763.
29. Sheriar N, Joshi R, Mukherjee Pal B, Birla A, Ray SK. Impact of structured counseling on the selection of hormonal contraceptive methods: results of a multi-centric, observational study in India, J Obstet Gynaecol India. 2014;64(4):241-50.
30. Mills AM, Wilkinson CL, Bromham DR, Elias J, Fotherby K, Guillebaud J, et al. Guidelines for prescribing combined oral contraceptives. BMJ. 1996;312(7023):121-2.
31. Burkman R, Schlesselman JJ, Zieman M. Safety concerns and health benefits associated with oral contraception. Am J Obstet Gynecol. 2004;190(Suppl):S5-22.
32. Redmond GP, Olson WH, Lippman JS, Kafrissen ME, Jones TM, Jorizzo JL. Norgestimate and ethinyl estradiol in the

treatment of acne vulgaris: a randomized, placebo-controlled trial. Obstet Gynecol. 1997;89:615-22.
33. IARC Working Group on the Evaluation of Carcinogenic Risks to Humans. Combined Estrogen-Progestogen Contraceptives and Combined Estrogen-Progestogen Menopausal Therapy. IARC Monographs on the Evaluation of Carcinogenic Risks to Humans Volume 91. Lyon, France: International Agency for Research on Cancer; 2007. pp. 74-84.
34. Heinemann LAJ, Dinger JC. Range of published estimates of venous thromboembolism incidence in young women. Contraception. 2007;75:328-36.
35. FSRH. (2017). FSRH Clinical Guideline: Contraception for Women Aged Over 40 Years. [online] Available from: https://www.fsrh.org/documents/fsrh-guidance-contraception-for-women-aged-over-40-years-2017/ [Last accessed January, 2024].
36. Appleby P, Beral V, Berrington de González A, Colin D, Franceschi S, Goodhill A, et al.; International Collaboration of Epidemiological Studies of Cervical Cancer. Cervical cancer and hormonal contraceptives: collaborative reanalysis of individual data for 16,573 women with cervical cancer and 35,509 women without cervical cancer from 24 epidemiological studies. Lancet. 2007;370:1609-21.
37. World Health Organization. Medical Eligibility Criteria for Contraceptive Use: A WHO Family Planning Cornerstone, 4th edition. Geneva: World Health Organization; 2010.

CHAPTER 24

Accelerating Quality Family Planning Services in the Private Sector in India: A FOGSI FWC Commitment

Shobha N Gudi, Radhika Chetan

INTRODUCTION

India has a rich history of efforts for family planning(FP)over7decadessince1952,mainly driven by public sector through implementation of focused programs. As a result, we do see steady improvement in the replacement level fertility rates with accelerated uptake of modern contraceptive methods (mCPR). The FP 2030 vision document (Government of India-August 2022) clearly demands innovative models for public and private sector partnership. It is indeed imperative that coordinated efforts by both sectors will ensure universal and reliable access to sexual and reproductive health especially for the vulnerable youth, considering India has the largest young population in the world. The National Family Health Survey (NFHS)-5 tells us that mCPR in the private sector has increased from 12 to 20% approximately.

World Health Organization (WHO) defines the private sector as: *"The private health sector is the individuals and organizations that are neither owned nor directly controlled by governments and are involved in provision of health services. It can be classified into subcategories as for profit and not for profit, formal and informal, domestic and international".*

COMPONENTS OF FAMILY PLANNING IN THE PRIVATE SECTOR

Components of family planning in the private sector is depicted in following.

FP products	Importers and manufacturers	Commercial and social marketing organizations	Supply chain (stockists, distributers, retailers, pharmacies)
FP information and training	Training institution—private medical and nursing colleges, etc.	Civil society organizations—NGOs, etc. —which build capacity of providers at various levels, create community awareness, demand generation, etc.	
FP service delivery	Service providers: • Social franchising networks • Clinics • Pharmacies • Secondary and tertiary care institutions	Online service providers: • Virtual clinics, inculding digital platforms like practo • E-pharmacies • Start-ups/social enterprises—ThatMate, etc.	

QUALITY IN FAMILY PLANNING SERVICES

It is defined as "Meeting the patient's needs and exceeding their expectations". Evidence suggests that the *quality family planning services have great impact on* uptake, continuation, and prevalence of contraception.[1,2]

The Elements of Quality Care in Contraception[2-5]

- Basket of choice of methods
- Information provided to clients
- Service provider technical competence and needs
- Interpersonal relations (client-provider interaction)
- Continuity of care
- Appropriate constellation of services.

Choice of Methods

- When one additional method is made available in the FP choice basket, it increased modern contraceptive use by 4–8 percentage points, based on 27 years of data for 113 countries.[3]
- World Health Organization recommends the choices in FP should include, a range of emergency, short-acting, long-acting, and permanent methods (SARC, LARC, EC, and limiting methods).
- Increasing the choices leads to increased uptake and increased continuation, allows flexibility, switching, overcomes method stockouts and ensures availability.

Information Provided to Clients

- Knowledge conveyed about available contraceptive methods including how to use, benefits and risks/potential side effects is important aspect of quality care.
- Improves—increased uptake of contraception due to dispelled myths and misconceptions, and increased continuation rates.

FOGSI-specific IEC material will go a long way in improving uptake in private sector.

Service Provider Technical Competence

- Quality needs command on the subject—Knowledge and skills of service provider needs to be increased by training and skill practice, clever use of MEC wheel
- *Higher procedural skills:* Reduced risk of infection and improper placement of subdermal implants and intrauterine devices and reduced complications in tubectomies and vasectomies.
- *Provider's needs:* Often neglected—frequent assessments for continuous supplies, adequate backup, referral for the complicated cases, feedback and acknowledgment of services, and payment of service dues if any.

Interpersonal Relations (Client-provider Interaction)

- Emphasis on verbal and nonverbal communication while counseling clients.
- Increased uptake and continuation due to being treated with *dignity and respect and approach with honesty, sympathy and understanding.*

Continuity of Care

- Establishing when and how clients will return to clinic, enhances satisfaction rates.
- Leads to decreased fertility rates due to increased contraceptive continuation rates/Decreased unwanted pregnancy.

Appropriate Constellation of Services

- Making contraception readily available to clients regardless of where they access care
- Increased access to contraception via service integration, integrated contraception clinics on the OPD floor of every obstetric unit
- Community outreach and mobile delivery of services
- Teleconsultation platforms linked to online pharmacy are promising options for the youth especially.

I-CARE BY FOGSI FAMILY WELFARE COMMITTEE (2019–22)

Among the private sector led initiatives there are few successful models, e.g., FOGSI concept of I-care which aimed at integrated contraceptive approach across reproductive ages. I-care clinics are the dedicated FP units to create an interphase between the couple and the healthcare worker. The overall concept is to utilize various platforms of care, for example:

- Adolescent care with contraceptive awareness.
- Preconceptional care with concept of reproductive planning
- Antenatal care to be strengthened by integrating counseling for postpartum contraception
- Postpartum care to be firmly ingrained with counseling and uptake for postpartum contraception.
- Comprehensive abortion care for postabortal contraception provision
- Premenopausal women coming in for gynecological care for checking and counseling on her contraceptive need.
- Integration with other services such as immunization, ICTC/PPTCT, RTI/STI clinic, mental healthcare, etc.

The presence of the private sector in India cannot be undermined as it consists of 58% of the hospitals in the country, 29% of beds in hospitals, and 81% of doctors.[6] Recent National Family Health Survey (NFHS-5) reveals that the private sector is one of the important sources for provision of modern contraceptives. Private sector contributes to 45% share of pills and 40% share of condoms. For other reversible contraceptives like injectables the share is 30% and for IUCD it is 24%. Sterilization services, however, are largely provided by the public sector in India.

The graph below shows that the contribution of the public sector has increased from 2015–16 to 2019–21 especially for all reversible modern methods **(Fig. 1)**. This necessitates the need for devising strategies to improve private sector engagement.

A clear shift has been observed where data for NFHS-5 is available (2019–20) toward increased use of reversible modern contraceptive methods across the country, and except for IUCD, most of the other reversible modern contraceptive methods were obtained from the private sector.

This data highlights that private sector will play an important role in addressing the equity gaps and ensuring access to family planning.

More than half of the poorest reversible contraceptive users rely on the private sector. Fifty-six percent (56%) of the poorest urban and 51% of the poorest rural users of reversible contraceptives obtain their method from a private sector source.

Private sector services seem to have contributed to the increase in contraceptive prevalence (for condom and pills); private nonmedical sources have been the greatest contributor.

The NFHS-5 data also indicate a significant rural urban gap. 48% urban and 38% rural population relies on the private sector for

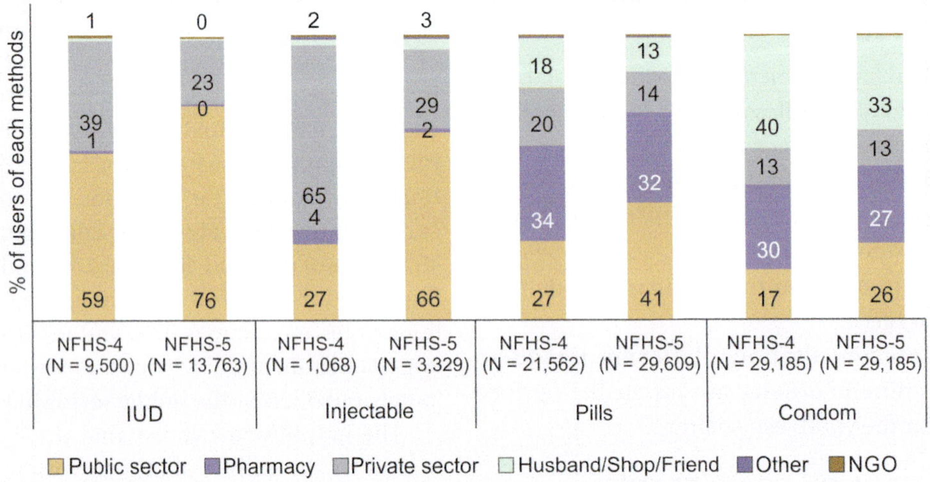

Fig. 1: Source of modern contraceptive. (NFHS: National Family Health Survey)

condoms. For pills also 56% urban and 41% rural population prefers private sectors. As the country is witnessing an increase in urbanization the gap may rise in future, again necessitating the need for engaging the private sector for contraceptive provision.

The demographic changes in the country will result in change age structure. India has the highest cohort of young people. When the young people use contraception, they go for reversible contraceptive methods and most get those from private sector. With the generational shift as younger people are more likely to access FP from the private sector in India, researchers also found low contraceptive knowledge (especially with regard to specific knowledge about contraception and methods).

STRATEGIES TO IMPROVE PRIVATE SECTOR PARTICIPATION FOR FAMILY PLANNING: CHARTING ROADMAP FOR 2030

India's large private sector has diversified role in augmenting services and demand for family planning. The current strategic approaches in the country follow different types of private sector engagements in India **(Fig. 2)**.

All the above strategic approaches are guided by a *supportive policy environment* and aim toward strengthening *access, quality, financing, commodity security* for "family planning".

Supportive Policy Environment

Implementing uniform policies across the states is a challenge as India has a large and complex private healthcare market. The government policy for empanelment aims at harnessing the private sector participation to its fullest. Though accreditation of private hospitals, clinics, and empanelment of practitioners through the state-driven programs are in place in many states through government regulatory models, enthusiasm by practitioners to participate for the same is not up to expectation.

Improving access to Family Planning Services

Various existing Public-Private Partnership models played a vital role in addressing

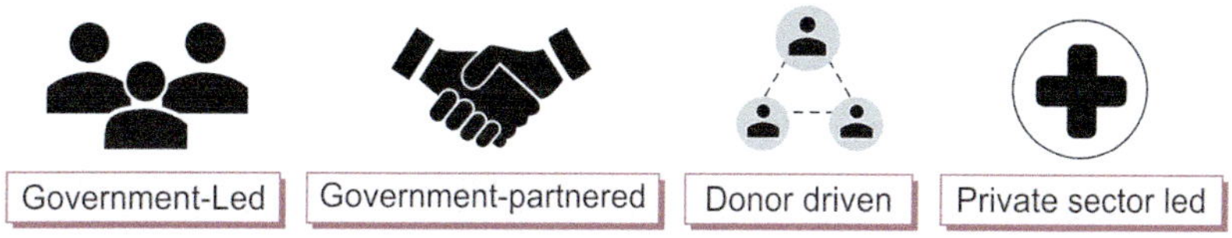

Fig. 2: Charting roadmap for 2030: different types of private sector engagements in India.

accessibility and affordability. Family Planning Division of the Ministry of Health and Family Welfare (MoHFW) insists on implementing the models of PPP, working in close collaboration with various national agencies, UN organizations, international funding agencies, professional bodies such as FOGSI, national and international NGOs, and the civil society, with the objective to enhance technical expertise and provide efficient services with equity.

Accreditation and Empanelment of Private Providers

India was an early starter in terms of implementing the clinic approach. Accreditation and empanelment of private and NGO facilities is a way to monitor quality, address the provider dearth and facilitate greater coordination with the private sector. The strategy works on mutual benefit whereby the private facility gets cover for the FP service provision and protection under government's indemnity scheme; the public system on other hand is able to address dearth of skilled human resource and logistics while the client gets a wider choice for availing FP services at free of cost. Presently, the accreditation and empanelment of private providers is limited to sterilization and IUCD services under National Family Planning Program.

Social Franchising for Family Planning: Social Franchising

Social franchising is a strategy to efficiently expand access to high-quality healthcare that is affordable to underserved populations (PSI, 2014). Social franchises are: Outlets (e.g., NGOs, clinics, pharmacies, mobile clinics) run by a network of service provider (e.g., midwives, nurses, doctors, pharmacists, and community health workers) where services are standardized and quality-controlled. Social franchising in FP/RH has been used to expand access to high-quality, affordable family planning services.

A social franchise is a network of private-sector healthcare providers that are linked through agreements to provide socially beneficial health services under a common franchise brand.

While strategizing for FP 2020 India identified the need for institutionalizing these innovative models and running the government partnered model. FP 2030 will provide a platform to plan, strategize, and institutionalize these models.

MISSION PARIVAR VIKAS SCHEME

Government's flagship program—Mission Parivar Vikas Scheme tried to address the service access issues in the seven challenged states. A special scheme for engaging with private provider was carved in 2016 whereby the private providers from adjacent districts were encouraged to provide FP services during Mission Parivar Vikas Campaigns (four times in a year). The special financial package was devised to cover the mobility and incidental cost for the private provider.

SOCIAL MARKETING OF CONTRACEPTIVES: SOCIAL MARKETING

Social marketing (SM) in family planning uses commercial marketing concepts to promote healthy behaviors and provide contraceptive products and services at subsidized rates, mostly in low-income communities (PSI, 2014; O'Sullivan et al., 2007). Uses marketing lens to develop strategies around the 4 Ps of *P*roduct, *P*rice, *P*lace, and *P*romotion. India was the first country to initiate the social marketing program for contraceptives, which started in 1968 with the launch of "Nirodh" (condom brand). Based on the total market approach, Government of India successfully partners with SMO (social marketing organizations) for provision of accessible and affordable modern contraceptive products. Subsequently, oral contraceptive pills were added in 1987. Government provides contraceptive products to SMOs at subsidized rates. SMOs are also given flexibility to promote both government as well as own branded products and services. SM platforms are a novel way of PPP.

EXPANDING CONTRACEPTIVE BASKET

Role of the private sector has been well acknowledged for the expansion of contraceptive baskets. This role extends from product manufacturing, research, marketing, and service provision. Often the introduction of new contraceptives in national programs is preceded by its introduction in private sector. Fulfilling its 2020 commitment India introduced two new contraceptives—Injectable MPA and Centchroman. The expansion and roll out utilized the experiences of the products in private sector market. The other methods new in contraceptive private sector are the etonogestrel implant, ulipristal acetate as emergency contraceptives, newer pills, IUDs, and LNG-IUS, and finally the SC-DMPA.

Strengthening Health Financing for Improved Outcomes

India significantly increased the resource envelope for improving FP services. The main strategic intervention for achievement of FP 2020 goals was to mobilize funds for ensuring private sector engagement. While striving to achieve FP 2020 goals, the country invested in accreditation and empanelment of private providers.

In addition, large donor investments were also diverted to augment private sector engagement.

Few of the donor led state innovations came up as best practice in India. The Hausla Sajhedari model (funded by BMGF) (implemented in Uttar Pradesh) provided a single window solution for easing the financial payments, accreditation, and empanelment process.

ASSESSMENT OF QUALITY: INDICATORS[7,8]

- Number of contraceptive methods available at a specific outlet.
- Percentage of counseling sessions with new acceptors in which provider discusses all methods.
- Percentage of client visits during which provider demonstrates skill at clinical procedures, including asepsis.
- Percentage of clients reporting "sufficient time" with provider
- Percentage of clients informed of timing and sources for re-supply/revisit
- Percentage of clients who perceive that hours/days are convenient and the range of services provided is adequate.

New Initiatives under Family Planning—Government of India (GOI)[9]

1. *Mission Parivar Vikas:* To accelerate access to high-quality family planning choices based on information, reliable services, and supplies within the rights framework.
2. Unified software for FP logistics
   - To streamline FP logistics and supply chain management.
   - Web-based, App-based and SMS-based application
   - Instant access to stock information from National level to ASHA level
3. Expansion of contraceptive basket of choices
4. New contraceptive packaging
5. New FP media campaign.

TAKE HOME POINTS ON QUALITY IN CONTRACEPTION

- Provision of clients' chosen method
- Offering the client adequate information
- Treating clients courteously
- Training providers
- Readiness (e.g., a range of methods with no stock outs, trained providers).

CONCLUSION

Private Sector-is therefore a Critical Lever to Achieve Universal Access to Family Planning and FOGSI has a substantial role eventually in fulfilling FP 2030 to achieve SDG. It must be acknowledged in all honesty that for this goal to be achieved huge efforts must be made to engage providers in Government programs, also private sector must formulate parallel strategies to perform effectively in this field. Evidence shows that several challenges exist to encourage and engage private sector:

- Practitioners are unaware of basket of choice of methods with newer options.
- The services may get limited to product sales (and not enough about method information).
- Expense of services may become higher without reason.
- Public-private partnership models need to be remodeled to avoid dropouts due to delayed reimbursements, procedural burden, trust deficit, and no significant increase in footfall.

We must revamp and restructure to prevent these factors from becoming an impediment to FP-2030 vision. Development of innovative models to address these challenges is necessary, as India's youth currently and in future require a private sector health system as much as they require public health system for reproductive health services and goals.

REFERENCES

1. Assaf S, Wang W, Mallick L. Quality of care in family planning services in Senegal and their outcomes. BMC Health Serv Res. 2017;17:346. https://doi.org/10.1186/s12913-017-2287-z
2. World Health Organization (WHO), 2017. Quality of care in contraceptive information and services, based on human rights standards: a checklist for health care providers; ISBN 978-92-4-151209-1. [online] Available from https://apps.who.int/iris/bitstream/handle/10665/254826/9789241512091-eng.pdf [Last accessed November, 2022].
3. Ross J, Stover J. Use of modern contraception increases when more methods become available: analysis of evidence from 1982-2009. Glob Health Sci Pract. 2013;1(2):203-12.
4. World Health Organization (WHO). Ensuring Human Rights in the Provision of Contraceptive Information and Services. Geneva: WHO; 2014.
5. Bruce J. Fundamental elements of the quality of care: a simple framework. Stud Fam Plann. 1990;21:61-91.

6. Thayyil J, Jeeja MC. Issues of creating a new cadre of doctors for rural India. Int J Med Pub Health. 2013;3 (1):8.
7. Sass CJ, Yinger NV. Overview of Quality of Care in Reproductive Health: Definitions and Measurements of Quality; New Perspectives on Quality of Care: No. 1; Washington: Population Council; 2002.
8. Institute of Medicine (US) Committee on a Comprehensive Review of the HHS Office of Family Planning Title X Program; Stith BA, Wright CE. A Review of the HHS Family Planning Program: Mission, Management, and Measurement of Results. Washington (DC): National Academies Press (US); 2009. Appendix K, Measurement of Quality in the Title X Family Planning Program. [online] Available from https://www.ncbi.nlm.nih.gov/books/NBK215198/ [Last accessed November, 2022].
9. Mission Parivar vikas guideline; Family planning guidelines NHM, Government of India. [online] Available from: https://nhm.gov.in/New_Update-2021-22/FP/MPV/Mission_Parivar_Vikas_Guidelines.pdf [Last accessed November, 2022].

INDEX

Page numbers followed by *f* refer to figure and *t* refer to table.

G

H

I

J

K

L

M